Emily's
Vinegar Diet
Book

by Emily Thacker

Published by:

James Direct Inc

500 S. Prospect Ave.

Hartville, Ohio 44632

U.S.A.

Not For Resale

ISBN: 978-1-62397-035-2

Printing 12 11 10 9 8

Table of Contents

DEAR READER,

Thank you for your interest in this book and others in the series. Your response to my previous books has been phenomenal. THE VINEGAR BOOK has more than 3,000,000 copies in print, in many languages, and in more than a dozen countries!

Your many letters are a continuing encouragement. They are filled with kind words and examples of ways you, too, use vinegar and natural home remedies. My mail also contains many requests for information on how to use vinegar as a regular part of the diet and as an aid in controlling weight. And so, I have put this collection of special diet information, weight loss tips and nutritional guidelines together for you. My sources include both anecdotical accounts from regular vinegar users and helpful hints inspired by scientific studies at major medical centers.

EMILY'S VINEGAR DIET is a common sense approach to life, health and eating for optimum health. It is an attempt to share with you what others are doing and how you can combine common sense eating with old-time folk wisdom. And so, it should come as no surprise to you that researchers now say a super-low-calorie diet is usually nutrient deficient and can be particularly dangerous for the mature adult.

Gradual changes in the way you eat improve your health with the most lasting results. EMILY'S VINEGAR DIET does not encourage you to suddenly drop 5 - 15 pounds in a single week. This approach to weight usually results in regaining any weight lost because, when you lose weight too fast, you send your body into famine mode. It begins to conserve fat and can actually make you gain weight by increasing your hunger!

This vinegar diet encourages you to eat the food you want. You do not need to deprive yourself. I feel you can eat the same number of calories you now eat, lower your risk of developing diseases linked to poor nutrition, and still lose weight. The secret is using a complex biological process called "thermogenesis" to burn away unwanted fat. EMILY'S VINEGAR DIET is as easy as filling your plate and as simple as increasing your body's metabolic rate. And, you will keep the weight you lose off because you will be eating more wisely and moving more.

EMILY'S VINEGAR DIET is not intended as medical advice; it has not been prepared or reviewed by a medical practitioner. Moderation, common sense and old-time remedies have always been the key to successful living. But they cannot take the place of medical advice so, when you are sick, you should seek the guidance of a competent medical practitioner. For everyday healthy living you may want to try the vinegar diet. It is designed to help you gradually, permanently, normalize weight, optimize energy and be vital at any age. This plan works because "dieting," as the term is commonly used, is not the way to regulate weight. A good diet is!

All diets have side effects. Some can leave you exhausted and hungry. Because EMILY'S VINEGAR DIET features generous amounts of vegetables and fruits its side effects can include extra energy, healthier bones, lower cholesterol, less risk of cancer or high blood pressure, less depression and a newly invigorated immune system!

Healthy eating offers you the opportunity to regain a more vibrant, vital body, a clear mind and the true joy of living. Promise yourself you will begin today!

Emily

The Wonder of Vinegar – What Others Are Saying*

"I went down to 183 from 280 .... I wouldn't trade what I did for all the money in this entire country. I feel and look different, and I'm 78 .... I just wanted you to know what apple cider vinegar did for me." VS., Meridian, Mississippi

"I went on .... apple cider vinegar and honey in water 3 times a day. I dropped 30 pounds so fast it scared me!" J.G., Sibley, Illinois

"My husband and I drink apple cider vinegar with apple juice, grape juice and water every day (for stabilizing blood pressure and cholesterol)." J. G., Sibley, Illinois

"Enjoyed your book very much. I read the whole thing in one afternoon!" G. S., Jamestown, New York

"I just finished reading your vinegar book. I bought 4, 3 for gifts. I know and believe much of what you wrote. " F.H., Hayes, Virginia

"2 teaspoons vinegar in a glass of water and drink with each meal — this will help you to lose weight." B. N., Willmar, Minnesota

"I am 70 years old and have used these recipes all my life and they work. .... To lose weight, a teaspoon honey and a teaspoon apple cider vinegar in a cup of tea or decaffeinated coffee." M.B., Sissonville, West Virginia

"Just a note to thank you for this great book. I am taking vinegar and water before meals for weight control.... also its settled the diarrhea caused by irritable bowel syndrome. I'm really pleased as I've suffered quite a few years...." K.T., Victoria, Australia

"I have used the honey and vinegar recipe for weight loss .... Thanks a lot." M.T., Sauk City, Wisconsin

"I thoroughly enjoyed the book .... being of Creek Indian heritage, my grandmother used many of your cures. I have read it five times already and have started using the honey and vinegar morning and night to already lose one and a half inches in my waist in one and a half weeks." Z.L., Pensacola, Florida

"My nephew told me that his cholesterol was 282. .... I told him to take one ounce vinegar and one tablespoon honey and six ounces of water, twice a day. In two months his doctor checked his cholesterol, it was 201. I ordered the vinegar book for (him)." J.S., Cleveland, Ohio

"In 1959 .... I started using a tablespoon of vinegar and a tablespoon of honey in two ounces of water every day. .... I'm still with the daily use. My hair still hasn't turned gray and I'm now past 80. Still bowling three times a week and have a 153 average .... Love that vinegar!" V.C., Seattle, Washington

Testimonials are atypical they may not reflect your personal results. You may lose more; you may lose less.

Chapter One

Why Vinegar? Because It Works!

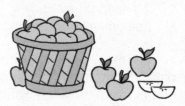

FOOD —

"Anything that sustains, nourishes and augments."

"Must contain in some form the actual chemical constituents of the new tissues which are being laid down."

DIET —

"A manner of living; food and drink habitually taken."

"Food prescribed for the prevention or cure of disease, or for attaining a certain physical condition."

VINEGAR IS PART OF A HEALTHY DIET! Vinegar has been used for centuries to aid health. Scientists tell us vinegar was probably part of the primordial soup of life. It is needed to burn fats and carbohydrates. The acid we know as vinegar is also used by the body as an aid in neutralizing poisons.

Often vinegar is combined with honey in a tonic that brings together the exceptional nutritional qualities of these two very special foods. Millions learned of this age-old tonic when its virtues were chronicled by physician D. C. Jarvis of Vermont. In Dr. Jarvis' book, FOLK MEDICINE, he praised the virtues of taking a daily tonic of apple cider vinegar and honey. His strong belief in the ability of apple cider vinegar to maintain an acid balance in the body was a large part of his faith in the tonic. His book stressed the common sense approach to food the Vermont country folk of his generation practiced. His "prescription" for maintaining health was to take, at least once a day:

Vinegar is good food.

2 Teaspoons apple cider vinegar
2 Teaspoons honey
Full glass of water

For those suffering from the pain of arthritis, rheumatism and other degenerative diseases he suggested the vinegar and honey combination be taken two to three times a day, with or before meals. Many people find a milder dose more palatable:

1 Teaspoon apple cider vinegar
1 Teaspoon honey
Full glass of water

DIET VS. DIETING

In recent times there has been an explosion of medical information. New ways of treating disease with drugs has driven food-based treatments into obscurity. The result, over the years, has been that much time-proven wisdom has been lost, forgotten or pushed aside. The notion that a well balanced diet was necessary for good health, as well as for weight control, was lost.

And so, my vinegar diet came into being! It is built around the fact that conventional "dieting" is not the best way to regulate weight and health. "Dieting" can be a dangerous health concept. It has come to mean a special, temporary way of relating to food that somehow turns a flabby, prematurely aged, malnourished body into a slim, trim, youthful one.

THIS IS BOTH UNTRUE AND UNFORTUNATE!

UNTRUE because it suggests a temporary change in eating can correct a lifetime of poor habits.

UNFORTUNATE because it leads to impossible expectations and almost ensures failure.

Throughout this volume I use the word "diet" to mean a lifelong way of nourishing a healthy body. It will not mean a temporary attempt to alter weight. Changes in body mass which come about by following the guidelines of the vinegar diet should be lasting, as well as promoting better health. It is a way to look better, feel better, be better!

DO YOU NEED THE VINEGAR DIET?

Does your present diet supply everything you need for optimum health? Ask yourself:

- Are you as healthy as you want to be?
- Are you as healthy as you ought be?
- Are you as healthy as you can be?

MOST DIETS ARE NUTRITIONALLY INADEQUATE! The typical diet does not supply enough of the nutrients needed for optimum health. It is estimated that less than 10% of the population follows the U.S. Agriculture Department's dietary guidelines. This means many do not get the Recommended Dietary Allowance (RDA) of important vitamins and minerals. And, the RDA gives only dietary minimums, the very smallest amount needed to prevent major diseases known to be caused by shortages. These amounts are not usually enough for maximum health.

RDA = Minimum amounts of vitamins and minerals, not optimal amounts!

Studies show more than half of those admitted to a hospital have a nutritional deficiency. The elderly are particularly at risk because, as the body ages it does not process foods as efficiently as it once did. And, the elderly tend to take more nutrient-depleting medications.

To extend the good years as long as possible means fighting the effects of degenerative diseases. Extra amounts of many nutrients can increase vitality and vigor, even in old age. But this can only be done by getting much more than the RDA of vitamins and minerals. The most frequently found nutrient shortages include:

Calcium	Magnesium	Thiamine
Chromium	Niacin	Vitamin A
Copper	Potassium	Vitamin B-12
Folic acid	Riboflavin	Vitamins C & D
Iron	Selenium	Zinc

DEFICIENCY SYMPTOMS

A low level of CALCIUM has been linked to depression and loss of bone mass. Foods high in phosphorus, such as meat and carbonated drinks, increase calcium loss, as do salt and caffeine.

Even marginally low levels of CHROMIUM can increase the risk of developing clogged arteries.

A body low on COPPER is more likely to get infections and some arthritis has been linked to unusual copper levels.

The likelihood of FOLIC ACID deficiency increases with age and can cause fatigue and increased susceptibility to infection.

Low iron is the most common nutritional deficiency.

Too little IRON is the most frequent cause of anemia and is associated with depression. It has even been linked to increased numbers of cold sores.

As many as 80% of senior citizens have at least marginally low levels of MAGNESIUM, which can cause diminished heart function and can be part of the cycle involved in angina pain.

The elderly, particularly those in institutions, frequently have lowered levels of NIACIN.

A low level of POTASSIUM is associated with depression, muscle weakness and fatigue.

Insufficient RIBOFLAVIN is associated with depression and increased susceptibility to infection, perhaps because it is needed to metabolize protein.

Too little SELENIUM has been linked to an increased risk of cancer and clogged arteries.

Slow healing of cuts and scrapes can be a sign of a shortage of THIAMINE, as can depression.

Those who do not get enough VITAMIN A are more likely to get infections.

Shortages of VITAMIN B-12 are linked to depression and excessive tiredness.

It is estimated that 40% of the women in the United States do not get enough VITAMIN C. Low vitamin C is associated with depression, tiredness and insufficient synthesis of collagen (which may encourage the advance of arthritis).

A shortage of VITAMIN D has been linked to bone loss and can result in arthritis doing damage to cartilage at a faster rate than it would otherwise.

Slow healing of cuts and scrapes and susceptibility to infection can be a sign of a shortage of ZINC. Its levels can be hurt by substances in eggs, milk and grains.

IS THERE A QUICK FIX?

Do I think taking mega-doses of vitamins and minerals head off or cure health problems? Not usually. Good nutrition is not that simple, because supplements can be risky. For example, everyone knows about the discomfort associated with too much acid in the stomach. But those with too little stomach acid are more susceptible to infections and parasites and are unable to properly absorb minerals such as calcium and iron. Only the proper balance aids digestion.

Individual metabolism determines the amount of a nutrient which can cause dangerous side effects. Anything which is a bit unusual about the way a body processes food can change a supplemental nutrient into a possibly life-threatening poison. Nutrients also need to be taken in proper proportion to each other because they interact in ways that are not yet fully understood. Researchers do know:

VITAMINS AND MINERALS CAN BE DANGEROUS IF TAKEN IMPROPERLY!

Too much CALCIUM can interfere with the body's supply of vitamin K or its absorption of zinc.

If the body's level of COPPER is too high, it is more likely to get

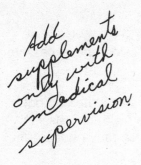
Add supplements only with medical supervision!

infections. Zinc levels can be lowered by copper, too.

Vitamin B-12 and zinc are compromised by too much FOLIC ACID.

Overdoses of IRON can result in liver damage, nausea and lowered levels of zinc and vitamin E.

Retaining too much MAGNESIUM is associated with depression. This mineral is depleted by a diet high in alcohol, caffeine, calcium and fat.

Flushing and itching are frequently associated with NIACIN supplementation.

Too much POTASSIUM interferes with the absorption of vitamin B-12.

Excess SELENIUM can cause diarrhea, hair loss, easily broken fingernails and garlicky smelling breath. Supplements are linked to a decrease in the risk of prostate, colorectal and lung cancer. But over supplementing can be fatal. It is hard to judge the amount of selenium in the diet because the natural content in food varies widely, depending on the soil where it was grown.

Itching and shortness of breath can be symptoms of excess THIAMINE.

Too much VITAMIN A increases fatigue symptoms, the risk of getting infections, headaches, brittle nails, and yellow tinted skin. The body needs plenty of vitamin A to repair cells and make strong scar tissue.

Extra VITAMIN B-12 can decrease feelings of tiredness and ease some allergic reactions of the skin, including itching. Too much can cause itching, too!

The body needs plenty of VITAMIN C to make strong scar tissue and to reduce the likelihood of getting infections. Some allergic reactions are dampened by extra vitamin C. Too much can cause diarrhea.

VITAMIN D helps the body use bone-building calcium. Too much can result in reduced kidney function as well as calcium deposits in joints and lungs.

When ZINC is elevated the immune response is dampened and copper absorption can be blocked. Extra zinc can decrease feelings of tiredness.

CAUTION: If you are taking mega-doses of nutrients — do not suddenly stop taking them. A body which has adjusted itself to a high level of a particular vitamin or mineral may react to an abrupt change by developing deficiency symptoms. ALWAYS consult with a medical professional before making changes to your normal routine!

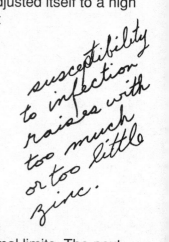

susceptibility to infection raises with too much or too little zinc.

POPPING PILLS IS NOT THE ANSWER

A good diet provides a generous supply of all the substances the body needs to maintain health and fight disease. There can be hundreds of important nutrients in a single serving of wholesome food. A good diet will also go a long way toward keeping weight within normal limits. The next chapter tells how to get balanced nutrients from food. And that is what the vinegar diet is about! It is a lifelong system of eating — a way of living — and a philosophy of health! Its principles can be the beginning of a new tomorrow of personal health for you.

EMILY SAYS

Vinegar, every day, is not for everyone. Many of my readers tell me vinegar is a tasty, beneficial, addition to their diets. Occasionally, a reader tells me the extra acid causes them some discomfort. YOU SHOULD NEVER CONTINUE EATING ANY FOOD THAT CAUSES DISCOMFORT WITHOUT DISCUSSING IT WITH YOUR HEALTH CARE PROVIDER! The beauty of my vinegar diet plan is that the principles of healthy eating, and the plate templates which show you how to eat foods in proportion to each other, can be used even if vinegar cannot be a regular part of your diet.

Chapter Two

Vinegar Magic

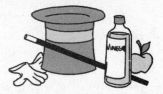

Good food contains more than the popular vitamins and minerals listed in most nutrient charts. In depth analysis of an ordinary apple reveals it contains more than 400 different substances! A single stalk of celery has nearly 450 identifiable components! Doctors do not yet know how the many substances in food work together in the body. They do know, when the body does not get everything it needs the result is sickness and wasting away of both tissue and bone. Even a marginal deficiency of a trace element or an essential nutrient can result in the body being unable to rebuild tissue and maintain the immune system.

THE MAGIC OF VINEGAR & HONEY

Since the most ancient of times people believed certain foods can have dramatic — even supernatural or miraculous — effects on health and well being. Vinegar and honey have been among these marvels, perhaps because they supply so many different nutrients.

APPLE CIDER VINEGAR A good, naturally produced vinegar contains far more than acetic acid. As apple juice ferments it produces a liquid laced with newly created alcohols, phenols and enzymes, while retaining tiny particles of apples with their storehouse of vitamins and minerals. Vinegar's enzymes are made by living bacteria. These enzymes are catalysts for biological reactions that are critical to life.

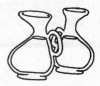

Along the way, vinegar picks up particles of other substances, too. Naturally processed vinegar is traditionally stored in wooden casks. This contributes to its virtues, as can be seen by the way its flavor is changed by the wooden barrels. The final result, that wonderful thing we call vinegar, has the goodness of the original food, plus much more!

HONEY Often, the concentrated flower power of honey is included in

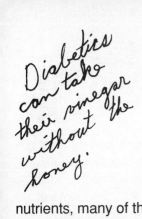
Diabetics can take their vinegar without the honey.

vinegar tonics. This rich sweetness is an ideal companion to vinegar's puckery tartness. Honey is nature's original sweetener. It contains an assortment of dissolved sugars such as sucrose, glucose and fructose. It also contains nearly 200 other substances, including minerals, vitamins, pigments, enzymes and amino acids.

Together, apple cider vinegar and honey provide a unique combination of health-promoting nutrients, many of them minute amounts of trace elements. Biochemists have now identified and measured hundreds of substances in the foods we eat. (Most nutrient charts list only the most plentiful and the most well known ones.) For a long time trace elements were ignored by most doctors and their importance to good health was underestimated.

Supplements are not the same as eating foods. The complex mix of phytochemicals in plants can not be duplicated chemically. And

Phyto = plant

so, multivitamin and mineral pills include only a very few of the substances known to be necessary for life. And, if too much of a vitamin or mineral is taken it can be stored in the body and end up as a poison. Extra nutrients that are not stored in the body must be filtered out by the kidneys, causing them to work harder than they otherwise would have to. The safest way to get the goodness of food is through healthy eating habits.

FORTIFIED VINEGARS

Fortified vinegars offer a way to combine the tremendous nutritional benefits of fruits and vegetables with the goodness of vinegar. Whole fruits and vegetables are used, so all their vitamins, minerals, enzymes and the hundreds of other components are preserved. They are an easy way to get a daily dose of vinegar. Fortified vinegars also perk up bland foods and — most of all — they are just plain good tasting!

Fortified vinegars begin with fruits and vegetables that are pureed in a blender with good, wholesome vinegar. Herbs and spices may be added, too. To prepare the recipes which follow, simply blend all ingredients until they are smooth and free of chunks.* The intensity of flavor which is best for you may vary from that of others. So, some optional seasonings are listed. Feel free to experiment with these recipes to produce your own personal variations. They make great dips, dressings for salads or marinades.

FORTIFIED APPLE CIDER VINEGAR & HONEY TONIC

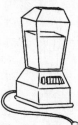

2   Medium apples
1/2 Cup apple cider vinegar
1/4 Cup honey

If you, like thousands of others, take a daily tonic of apple cider vinegar and honey, 1 tablespoon of this dressing is an especially appetizing way to do it! Optional ingredients: 1/2 teaspoon cinnamon, 1/4 teaspoon nutmeg and an additional 1/4 cup honey (if cinnamon is added). In addition to all the nutrients in apple cider vinegar and honey this combination adds the goodness of fresh apples. Included in the nearly 400 substances that have been identified in apples are:

- Calcium, beta carotene, carotenoids, chlorophyll, fiber, folacin, fructose, glucose, clycine, lecithin, lysine, pectin, niacin, selenium, sorbitol, sucrose, thiamin, tryptophan and zinc.

CUCUMBER-CELERY
1   Large cucumber
2   Cups celery
1   Cup red wine vinegar
1   Cup water

Good for seasoning steamed vegetables, boiled potatoes or pasta. Optional ingredient: 1/2 teaspoon salt. In addition to all the nutrients in vinegar this combination adds the goodness of fresh cucumbers and celery. Included in the nearly 450 substances that have been identified in celery and the more than 175 substances that have been identified in cucumbers are:

- Calcium, beta carotene, carotenes, choline, copper, coumarin, beta elemene, glycine, histidine, iron, lysine, riboflavin, tryptophan and tyrosine. (Celery)

- Beta amyrin, calcium, beta carotene, fluorine, folacin, iron, lysine, riboflavin, selenium, beta sitosterol, thiamin, tryptophan and tyrosine. (Cucumbers)

For maximum nutritional benefits, use immediately.

GARLIC

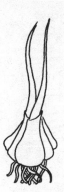

8   Garlic bulbs
1   Cup apple cider vinegar
    Bake fresh, whole garlic bulbs until tender. Peel
away the outer skin and squeeze the soft garlic paste
into a blender. Blend in the apple cider vinegar. Optional
ingredients: 1/2 to 1 cup oil, 1/2 to 1 teaspoon salt, 2
teaspoons sugar, 2 teaspoons dry mustard. In addition to all
the nutrients in vinegar this combination adds the goodness
of fresh garlic. Included in the more than 275 substances
that have been identified in garlic are:

- Ascorbic acid, calcium, beta carotene, copper, fiber, clycine,
  lysine, niacin, riboflavin, selenium and thiamin.

RASPBERRY

1   Cup raspberries
3   Tablespoons red wine vinegar
    Raspberries may be fresh or frozen, sweetened or unsweetened.
Great over ice cream, peaches, melon slices or fruit salad. In addition
to all the nutrients in vinegar this combination adds the goodness of
red raspberries. Included in the more than 100 substances that have
been identified in red raspberries are:

- Acetic acid, ascorbic acid, boron, calcium, beta carotene,
  chromium, fiber, lactic acid, pectin, riboflavin, salicylic acid,
  selenium, tannin and thiamin.

CUCUMBER-ONION

1   Large cucumber
1/2   Cup red wine vinegar
1/4   Cup onion
    No need to peel a well scrubbed cucumber or remove the seeds.
Optional ingredients: 1/4 to 1/2 cup oil or replace the red wine with
champagne vinegar. In addition to all the nutrients in vinegar and
cucumbers, this recipe adds the goodness of onions. Included in the
nearly 350 substances that have been identified in onions are:

- Ascorbic acid, calcium, beta carotene, choline, fiber, lysine,
  niacin, pectin, riboflavin, selenium and sulfur.

CARROT

1	Cup carrots
1/2	Cup apple cider vinegar
1/2	Cup water
3 to 4	Tablespoons honey (optional)

Use raw carrots for a cool vegetable dip, cooked ones for a smoother sauce to top cooked foods or add to soups. In addition to all the nutrients in vinegar this recipe adds the goodness of carrots. Included in the more than 400 substances that have been identified in carrots are:

Cooking carrots increases their beta carotene!

- Ascorbic acid, boron, calcium, citric acid, copper, glycine, lecithin, lysine, niacin, riboflavin, selenium, thiamin, tryptophan, vitamin B-6, vitamin D and vitamin E. Plus, carrots contain alpha, beta, epsilon and gamma carotenes.

Recipes for some other fortified vinegars which are packed with healthy phytochemicals follow:

STRAWBERRY

1	Cup strawberries
1/4	Cup champagne vinegar

This is a mildly tart vinegar that is high in vitamin C. Optional ingredients: 1/2 cup yogurt or 2 tablespoons honey.

HONEYDEW

2	Cups honeydew melon
1/4	Cup champagne vinegar
1/4	Cup water

Excellent topping for fruits and ices. Optional ingredients: 1 tablespoon honey or 1/4 teaspoon ginger.

BLUEBERRY

2	Cups blueberries
3/4	Cup red wine vinegar
3/4	Cup water

Use fresh or frozen berries. Optional ingredient: 2 tablespoons honey.

LEMON

1   Lemon
2   Tablespoons champagne vinegar
1/2   Cup water

    Use the entire lemon, both pulp and peeling. Excellent splashed on sea food. Optional ingredient: 1 cup cabbage.

Use fortified vinegars to get more fruits and vegetables into your diet.

PARSLEY

2   Cups fresh parsley
1/2   Cup red wine vinegar
1/2   Cup water

    This bright green vinegar goes well with meats and steamed vegetables.

KALE-MUSTARD

2   Cups kale, fresh or cooked
1/4   Cup apple cider vinegar
1/4   Cup water
2   Tablespoons dry mustard

    This is a thick and healthy dip or a topping for vegetables. Optional ingredient: 15 peppercorns.

MINT SAUCE

2   Cups fresh mint leaves
1   Cup apple cider vinegar
2   Tablespoons honey
   Malt or red wine vinegar may be substituted.

ARE YOU OVERFED & UNDERNOURISHED?

    Once it was thought good nutrition was only important for babies and growing children. Now we realize the adult body needs adequate amounts of protein, carbohydrates, vitamins, minerals — as well as hundreds of trace elements — to function properly and to retard premature aging. The best mix of these substances, and sometimes the only place they can be found, is in the foods supplied to the body. We now know that, for adults, fruits and vegetables are more important than ever!

    Yet, dietitians tell us it is almost impossible to get all needed nutrients from the foods most people eat. If the diet does not contain enough leafy green vegetables, the body may be short of the folic acid needed to protect it from heart attack and stroke. A shortage of a tiny amount of a trace element can affect the emotions. If vitamin E, such as is found in wheat germ is in short supply, the risk of developing Parkinson's and Alzheimer's diseases may rise. The selenium in foods such as garlic help fight cancer and the beta carotene in cantaloupe and carrots is an antioxidant that soaks up free radicals that age the body.

Free radical particles are left over from food digestion. These oxygen-rich substances damage body cells in the same way they make iron rust, vegetables rot and oils rancid. Free radicals can cause cells to lose their ability to function properly, or even die. Antioxidants such as flavonoids, carotenoids, vitamin C and vitamin E are the body's defense against free radicals. These protectives are found in fruits and vegetables. I have found that some very special things happen when lots of fruits and vegetables are added to the diet. They include:

- A daily dose of pectin (the amount found 2 or 3 apples) may be able to lower cholesterol — by as much as 25% or more.

- Even when a diet contains more fat than doctors feel is healthy, extra fruits and vegetables can help lower blood pressure. And the benefits begin in as little as two weeks!

- Adding garlic to the diet can reduce the likelihood of getting an infection. It fights 17 different kinds of fungus.

- Eating lots of both garlic and onion has been linked to lower levels of cholesterol.

- The carotenoid in tomatoes has twice the antioxidant power of beta carotene!

Chapter Three

The Vinegar Diet

CAN THE VINEGAR DIET BRING NEW HEALTH TO YOUR LIFE?

VERY PROBABLY!

Eating better with the vinegar diet is about a whole lot more than vinegar! It is a complete way of living and feeling better about yourself. And best of all, you can begin today. Eating better and feeling better is as simple as filling your plate! Never again count calories, weigh food or struggle with measuring cups. The vinegar diet is as easy as filling your plate, as pleasant as eating your favorite food, and as good for you as sunshine in the morning!

My vinegar diet combines what we have always instinctively known about eating with the best of the tips I have found in today's biochemical research. It is good food for a healthy body without:

- Confusing calorie counting.
- Complicated rules.
- Depressing restrictions.
- Fad foods.
- Expensive supplements.

Fifty years ago your Grandmother said, "Eat your fruits and vegetables." Twenty-five years ago your Mother said, "Eat your fruits and vegetables." Today's best scientific research confirms their wisdom. Best health only comes when you eat your fruits and vegetables!

Fruits and vegetables are the heart of healthy eating. And, many believe a daily vinegar tonic is also a good idea! Vinegar is an essential building block for the body. It can also help the body absorb the calcium it needs to ward off osteoporosis because calcium needs stomach acid to be absorbed well. Yet, many of those who desperately need calcium, those over 60, have reduced amounts of natural stomach acid.

EMILY'S VINEGAR DIET

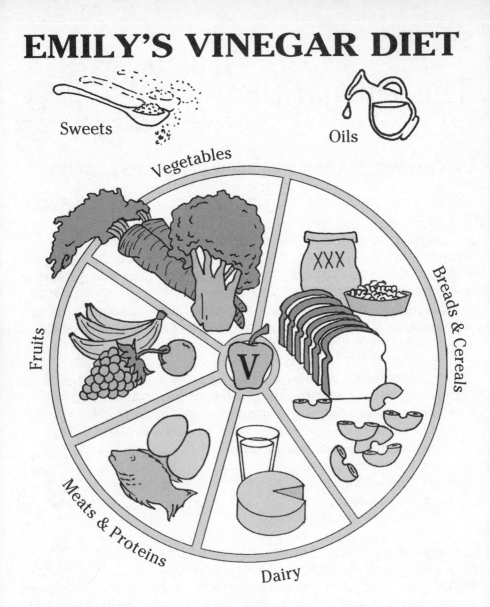

Sweets

Oils

Vegetables

Fruits

Breads & Cereals

Meats & Proteins

Dairy

EMILY SAYS

Use this drawing to eat food in the proper proportions. Every meal, and every snack, should contain something from each food group.

- Add sweets in moderation, especially refined sugars.
- Add oils in moderation, especially saturated fats.
- Dairy products are especially important, as they supply calcium for healthy bones.

THE VINEGAR DIET

Traditionally, vinegar and honey are taken with a full glass of water 30 minutes before the two largest meals of the day.* Taken this way they help control appetite, aid digestion and supply trace amounts of a spectacular number of nutrients. (If you take a vinegar tonic on a daily basis, use a straw so tooth enamel is protected.)

THE SECRET TO THE VINEGAR DIET IS PROPORTION!! Each time you eat, use the drawing on the opposite page. It shows you how much of each food group to eat at each meal. It is essential to use these proportions every time you eat! Every day, you need to include foods in your diet from all five food groups:

- Grains & breads - includes rice, potatoes, pasta, beans, baked goods.
- Vegetables - includes broccoli, squash, green beans, corn, tomatoes.
- Fruits - includes oranges, bananas, grapes, pears, berries, melons.
- Proteins - includes meat, fish, peanut butter, beans.
- Dairy - includes milk, yogurt, cottage cheese, buttermilk.

If you are eating a big meal and heap up lots of food on the bread and grain section, then you must also heap up lots of food on all the other sections. This way, the food you eat stays in proper proportion. If you go back for seconds, you must eat some of each food group, in the proportions shown. If you are only eating a snack, fill each section sparingly.

Add fats and sweets sparingly to the foods above and drink six to eight glasses of water a day. To maintain an average weight and to get the nutrients your body needs each day, you need:

- 6 to 11 servings of breads and grains
- 3 to 5 servings of vegetables
- 2 to 4 servings of fruits
- 2 to 3 servings of protein
- 2 to 3 servings of dairy products
- A few splashes of oil or fats
- A bit of sugar or sweets

Healthy goal = 30% (or less) calories from fat.

*See Chapter One

SAMPLE MEALS

Breakfast:

Breads and grains	Bagel
Vegetables	Tomato
Fruit	Cantaloupe
Protein	Peanut butter
Dairy	Yogurt

Full meal:

Breads and grains	Pasta and a dinner roll
Vegetables	Green beans and beets
Fruits	Orange
Protein	Fish
Dairy	Skim milk

Light meal:

Breads and grains	Rice
Vegetables	Broccoli and carrots
Fruits	Grapes
Protein	Chicken
Dairy	Skim milk

Snack:

Breads and grains	Crackers
Vegetables	Cucumber
Fruits	Cherries
Protein & dairy	Cottage cheese

Make sure the amount of food for each food group fits inside the space allotted for it. Each helping must fit on its place on the sample plate. If the total amount is more food than you want, adjust the size of portions rather than allowing yourself to skip an entire food group.

 For example, if an entire plateful of breakfast is more food than you want, serve yourself 1/2 a bagel, a couple of cherry tomatoes, a small sliver of cantaloupe, a teaspoon of peanut butter and 1/4 cup of yogurt. If you want a hearty breakfast, serve yourself an entire bagel, a large tomato, 1/2 a cantaloupe, a tablespoon of peanut butter and a cup of yogurt.

Occasionally, one section of a meal may overlap another. When this happens, make up for it at the next meal. For example, if a piece of fish overlaps its section at one meal, you may skip the protein section on the next meal and fill that area with extra vegetables or fruits. And remember, many kinds of beans can do double duty because they are good sources of protein.

Keep fats and oils to a minimum by trimming meats and avoiding fried foods. Limit sugar and sweets by replacing them with fruits.

Fortified vinegars can help you increase the amount of vegetable and fruit nutrients you get. They are also good ways to get your daily servings of vinegar. For example, in the sample full meal, serve the fish topped with lemon or garlic fortified vinegar. In the sample snack, apple fortified vinegar is a smooth, tasty way to add flavor, nutrients and excitement to the cottage cheese.

COLOR MATTERS

Good food comes in a healthy rainbow of colors. Always look at your plate of food and check that you have included many different colors. If the plate is mostly white, faded and colorless your food is probably over-processed and short of nutrients. Your diet should be a joyful mix of color. Check for a variety of colors at every meal, every day. Include foods that are red, orange, yellow, purple and green because:

• Red foods can contain lycopene that fights cancer; others have betacyanin that fights bacteria. Red foods include radishes, tomatoes, strawberries, cherries, raspberries, grapes, peppers, beans, watermelon, cranberries, beets and apples.

• Orange foods can contain beta carotene, which lowers the risk of getting some cancers. Orange foods include squash, carrots, oranges, pumpkins, sweet potatoes, cantaloupe, papayas and apricots.

• Yellow foods can contain lutein to help preserve eyesight by fighting macular degeneration. Others have the antioxidant anthoxanthin, or an anti-inflammatory, antibacterial and antiviral substance called quercetin. Yellow foods

For best antioxidant action eat colorful foods.

include raspberries, cherries, peppers, grapefruit, squash, lemons, corn, beans, bananas, pineapple and apples.

- Purple foods can contain anthocyanin, a phytochemical that attacks free radicals while also dilating blood vessels to reduce the risk of stroke and heart attack. Purple foods include egg plant, red cabbage, blackberries, raspberries, grapes, blueberries, cherries and plums.

- Green foods can contain indoles that block some cancer causing chemicals. Green foods include broccoli, Brussels sprouts, kiwis, grapes, peppers, spinach, beans, apples, asparagus, celery, kale, okra and cucumbers.

BOOST THE HEALTH EFFECTS OF THE VINEGAR DIET!

You can multiply the benefits of my vinegar diet by drinking six to eight glasses of water each day and limiting coffee to one or two cups. Take an energy boosting "mini vacation" of 10 minutes from your usual day. Get outside into the fresh air. Move around a bit, let your mind wander. Never skip meals. Eat several small meals instead of one or two large ones that can make you feel sluggish and bloated. Give yourself a new routine by making changes in the way you do things during the day.

Learn to reward yourself in nonfood ways. Have a massage instead of dinner at a fancy restaurant. You will feel better, longer. Do some deep breathing exercises instead of eating a handful of cookies. Move around more to improve circulation. Wear brightly colored, soft comforting clothes. Sit in the sunshine, outside when the weather is nice, at a window when weather is bitter. But most important, begin right this minute! Put a smile on your face, think about something pleasant, and vow to yourself that you are going to begin eating for health with the next bite you take by following the vinegar diet plan!

VINEGAR DOES EVEN MORE

One of biggest jobs vinegar does in the human body is promote the growth of beneficial bacteria. They are needed to keep disease-producing germs at bay. For example, human intestines contain millions of good bacteria (such as bifidus and lactobicillus) to keep the gastrointestinal tract healthy and disease free. Helpful bacteria in the intestines also work to:

- Support the immune system.
- Help digest food.
- Make some vitamins.
- Keep the intestines acidic.
- Discourage illness caused by E. coli and clostridia bacteria.

Easy on the salt.

Fruits and vegetables are storehouses of flavonoids, biflavonoids and carotenoids. These are wondrous antioxidants with the ability to neutralize free radicals that age the body. Of the hundreds of flavonoids in plants, more than 60 kinds (such as beta carotene) have been found in the foods we eat. For example, you can get your entire daily beta carotene needs in half a cantaloupe or half a carrot. The cantaloupe has the vitamin C of two small oranges.

CHOLESTEROL

Almost all body cells have some cholesterol. The body makes some, and it is found in all animal-based foods. Meat, fish, poultry, eggs and dairy products all have it. Some cholesterol is essential. The body uses it to build new cells, make hormones and as an aid in digestion. Too much contributes to clogging arteries and heart damage.

Vegetables, which are cholesterol free, are a very healthy way to get protein. Cold water fish help maintain low cholesterol, too. They bring cholesterol lowering omega-3 fatty acids to the body. (This is probably because of the way omega-3 fatty acids act on platelet aggregation and lipid metabolism.)

FIBER

Vegetables and fruits bring fiber to the diet. Fiber helps regulate digestion, absorbs cholesterol and dilutes toxins that cause cancer. Foods containing soluble fiber include rye, oats, legumes and fruits such as apples. Food containing insoluble fiber include whole wheat, bran and most fruits and vegetables.

Thermogenics food becomes heat + energy.

CARBOHYDRATES

High doses of sugar hurts cells' ability to fight disease. Complex carbohydrates in fruits and vegetables stay in the digestive system longer, and are fed into the blood stream more slowly than refined sugars. This slow, steady digestion keeps essential nutrients in the bloodstream. They bathe cells in healing antioxidants for long periods of time. A cell which is bathed in nutrients will go a long way in healing itself.

A low fat, sugar and cholesterol diet may be helpful in fighting infection. So is eating enough protein. The risk of many chronic diseases of elder years is increased by poor eating habits in younger years. And poor nutrition makes recovery from illness take longer.

THERMOGENESIS — A WORD YOU NEED TO KNOW

Thermogenesis is the process by which the body turns food into energy. This energy is used to warm the body, make muscles work and power the brain. And, some is used to repair and replace worn out tissue. When you eat, think about what kind of nutrients that particular food is giving your body. If it is a very fatty food it may supply more energy than the body can work off, without giving it the vitamins and minerals it needs to repair injury. The result is fat added to the body.

FOOD MYTHS

- There are no calories in cottage cheese.
- Pickles and milk at the same meal will make you sick.
- Bread sticks have very few calories.
- Brown eggs are better than white eggs.
- Ice cream is the secret to losing weight.
- Hot food is healthier than cold food.

Good health and a youthful appearance go hand in hand with a good diet. It has been said that the body's real age is tied closer to the health of its immune system than to its calendar age. I believe nutritious food and moderate exercise are the best ways to empower the immune system, to bring a healthy glow to your face and to put a spring into your step. You can improve your appearance by feeding your body everything it needs. This includes eating a wide variety of foods.

Promise yourself you will begin today to make better choices.

ET SAYS   IS THE VINEGAR DIET FOR YOU?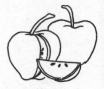

Ask your doctor before beginning any changes to your usual diet. The suggestions offered in The Vinegar Diet may be appropriate for healthy adults — they are not intended for children, the frail elderly, those taking medications or with chronic health conditions — without the approval of a medical professional!

Chapter Four

Lose Weight The Vinegar Way

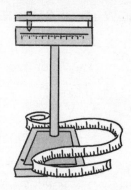

CAN VINEGAR MELT AWAY POUNDS AND INCHES? Doctors tell us when calories are restricted as a way to lose weight 95% of diets fail! Harsh dieting, with strict calorie reduction, is harmful to the body and an unnatural process. When you are hungry the natural thing to do is eat! Strict "dieting" can affect the immune system, making it unable to do a good job fighting off disease. People who spend a lifetime gradually putting on pounds should not expect to take it all off overnight.

SO, CAN YOU REALLY USE MY VINEGAR DIET TO MELT FAT AWAY?

YES!

There is a way for you to eat all the food you need to feel full and create the slimmer body you have always wanted! If weight loss makes you look drawn and ill you are losing weight too fast. Losing weight is a very complex process. You can win the war against unwanted pounds, but it is important to not lose important nutrients along with the weight.

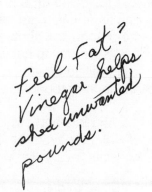

feel Fat? Vinegar helps shed unwanted pounds.

What is the very best diet of all? The one that works for you — the vinegar diet plan! It can help you keep off unwanted pounds for life. Its slow and steady weight loss means you never need to "go on a diet" again. You will feel better about yourself and have more energy from the very beginning. It is a way of living, a plan for a healthier life!

HOW TO BE THINNER, LOOK YOUNGER, FEEL MORE VIGOROUS!

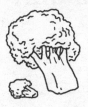 Depriving yourself of food, being constantly hungry or even having to count calories is not the way to create a healthy new body. To begin using the vinegar diet to help you lose weight, review vinegar and honey use in Chapters One, Two and Three. Follow my vinegar diet eating plan at every meal and every time you eat a snack.

THE SECRET TO LOSING WEIGHT WITH THE VINEGAR DIET IS PROPORTION!! Each time you eat, use the drawing on the opposite page. It shows you how much of each food group to eat at each meal. It is essential to use these proportions every time you eat! And, just as in the regular vinegar diet, you must include foods from all five food groups in your diet each day:

Grains & breads... includes rice, potatoes, pasta, beans, baked goods.
Vegetables........... includes broccoli, squash, green beans, corn, tomatoes.
Fruits................... includes oranges, bananas, grapes, pears, berries, melons.
Proteins .... includes meat, fish, peanut butter, beans.
Dairy .... includes milk, yogurt, cottage cheese, buttermilk.

Resist the urge to pile up your plate with huge amounts of food at one time. If you are very hungry, fix a medium-sized plate of food using the proportions shown on my vinegar weight loss diet plate. Then wait a few minutes to decide if you are really hungry for more food. If you are, refill your plate, being sure to select food from each food group and in the proportions shown.

Add fats and sweets very sparingly and drink at least eight glasses of water a day. Even if you are determined to lose weight as rapidly as possible, every day your body needs at the very least:

- 4 to 6 servings of breads and grains
- 3 to 4 servings of vegetables
- 3 to 4 servings of fruits
- 2 to 3 servings of protein
- 2 to 3 servings of dairy products
- A splash of oil or fat
- A sprinkle of sweetness

EMILY'S VINEGAR WEIGHT LOSS DIET

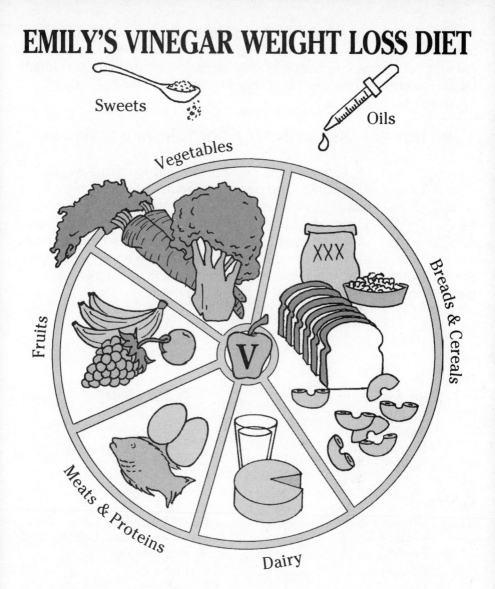

EMILY SAYS

Use this drawing to eat food in the proper proportions. Every meal, and every snack, should contain something from each food group.

- Add sweets sparingly, especially refined sugars.
- Add oils sparingly, especially saturated fats.
- Low fat dairy products are especially important, as they supply calcium for healthy bones.

You need to eat at least the number of servings of each food group listed above every day. Any less food and your body will be at risk for a nutrient deficiency. Depending on the foods you choose and how much fat and sweets you add, this diet should provide you with between 1200 and 1600 calories.

DO NOT EAT LESS WITHOUT A DOCTOR'S SUPERVISION!

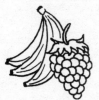

Limiting fat is the simplest way to control weight. As a bonus, you decrease the risk of stroke, high blood pressure and diabetes. Your goal, for the most successful, longest lasting weight loss is to begin your vinegar diet by keeping the number of calories you eat each day about the same as you are eating right now. Simply switch fat calories to calories from fruits and vegetables and begin to increase the amount of exercise you get.

SAMPLE MEALS

Breakfast:
Breads and grains	Puffed wheat
Vegetables	Tomato
Fruit	Cantaloupe
Protein	Slice of turkey breast
Dairy	Skim milk

Full meal:
Breads and grains	Sweet potato
Vegetables	Green beans, beets, salad
Fruits	Orange, kiwi
Protein	Fish
Dairy	Skim milk

Light meal:
Breads and grains	Rice
Vegetables	Broccoli, carrots
Fruits	Grapes, apple
Protein	Chicken
Dairy	Yogurt

Snack:

      Breads and grains............................ Crackers
      Vegetables....................................... Cucumber, celery
      Fruits.. Cherries, grapefruit
      Protein & dairy .... Cottage cheese

Make sure the size of each helping of food fits on its place on the sample plate. Compared to my standard vinegar diet, the vinegar weight loss diet gives you slightly smaller portions of breads and grains and slightly larger portions of vegetables and fruits. The protein and dairy sections are exactly the same. If the diet seems to offer more food than you want, adjust the size of portions rather than skip an entire food group.

For example, if breakfast is more food than you want to eat, serve yourself 1/2 cup of cereal, a couple of cherry tomatoes, a small sliver of cantaloupe, a very small piece of turkey and a glass of skim milk. If you are very hungry, serve yourself a full cup of cereal, a large tomato, 1/2 a cantaloupe, a small slice of turkey and drink a full glass of skim milk.

If a food does overlap one section, make it up at the next meal. For example, if a piece of fish overlaps its section at one meal, you may skip the protein section at the next meal and fill that area with extra vegetables or fruits.

LOSE POUNDS – THE VINEGAR WAY

As you can see, the vinegar weight loss diet is very similar to the regular vinegar diet. And that is the magic of this eating plan! You lose weight by eating extra vegetables and fruits and increasing how much you move around. This makes it an amazing – perhaps the ultimate – weapon against fat!

To the body most "diets" seem like a deadly famine.

You will protect the health of your heart and arteries, and lose weight, by eating very small amounts of fats and oils. Limit sugars and sweets, too. Use fortified vinegars to increase the amount of vegetable and fruit nutrients you get, and as an alternative to drinking vinegar in water.

For example, in the sample breakfast the cantaloupe is delicious topped with fortified raspberry vinegar. In the sample light meal fortified carrot vinegar can be served over the broccoli. Or, spoon warm garlic fortified vinegar over both the broccoli and carrots.

Several times a week substitute legumes, such as beans, for animal sources of protein. Many kinds of beans do double nutritional duty because they are good sources of protein. You will eliminate cholesterol loaded fats and be able to eat much larger portions for the same calories. And, beans make you feel full for hours longer than many other foods. To use the plate diagram for plant-based sources of protein (such as beans) use both the bread and grain and protein sections when filling your plate.

THERMOGENESIS — A CONCEPT FOR LOSING WEIGHT

The body thinks of food as fuel. So, its first instinct is to turn it into energy. Some energy is used to power muscles and the brain. A lot of energy is used to heat the body and a tiny bit is used to replace worn out or damaged cells. Only after doing all this does the body make fat.

A diet that gives you a headache is too harsh.

If there is a sudden reduction in the amount of food the body gets it panics and thinks a famine has started. To protect itself from dying in this famine all available calories are turned into fat. And, worst of all, the body sends urgent signals of hunger to its appetite control center.

Little wonder many doctors tell us nearly all of the weight lost by conventional calorie reduction "dieting" is soon regained! The very best way to begin a weight loss program is to lower total body fat and increase lean body mass, while keeping actual weight steady. Muscle takes more calories to maintain, even at rest. This means the body uses more calories, so weight is gradually reduced, even though the amount of food eaten stays constant.

This thermogenic weight loss happens because muscles have a higher metabolic rate than fat. And, muscles weigh more than fat for the same bulk. So, for the same total weight, extra muscle means a slimmer body. And, increased muscle tone will enable you to have a firmer abdomen and stronger back muscles, which will make you appear slimmer. As more and more fat is replaced with muscle, the higher metabolic rate will need enough extra calories that the body will begin using up its stored fat.

The second part of thermogenic weight loss is based on the fact that the body's biggest use of calories is to make heat. What is left over goes to fix worn out body parts and allow muscles to do work. Only after all this is fat produced. If the cycle is interrupted anywhere along the way, there is no fat to store.

When fuel is low the body's thermostat is turned down.

Thermogenesis, turning food into heat, can be increased by diet choices. You can feel it begin when you eat a big meal and your body gets hot as it burns food. Some foods do this longer and better than others. They encourage the body to burn calories faster by increasing metabolism. By adding these foods to the diet and by moving around more you lose weight without reducing the total number of calories in the diet. Healthy, fat-free fortified vinegars (like all foods) get the process of thermogenesis to begin working for you.

If you suddenly restrict calories, the body slows down its metabolic rate. Food is stored as fat instead of being used as energy. When the rate of metabolism is high, more food is burned and less is available to make fat. (When the rate of metabolism is very low it is almost impossible to lose weight, even on a severely restricted calorie diet.) Cold, food and exercise speed up thermogenesis. Increasing the number of calories the body burns is a sure, safe and lasting way to lose weight.

COLD When the body is chilled, it has to work harder and burn more calories to keep warm. That is why I believe cooling off the body helps increase its metabolic rate. For example, always wearing a heavy sweater could help the body stay fat by reducing the amount of calories it needs to burn to stay warm.

EXERCISE Exercise turns up the body's fat-burning metabolism. This faster burning of calories continues for hours after exercise has ended. For this reason I suggest spreading exercise out over the entire day, rather than

I feel my fortified vinegars can promote thermogenesis.

limiting it to a single session. To practice this, get moving early in the day. Make your body wake up and begin using calories as soon as possible. Follow up with frequent short exercise periods.

FOOD Some foods, such as capsicum-containing peppers increase metabolism. They burn off more calories than they contain because they stimulate the body. Thermogenic agents such as hot peppers and chili powder also have lots of vitamins C and E, carotenes and antioxidants. They even have substances to fight the bacteria which causes some diarrhea. Fennel is another good "diet" food. Fennel can be of great help in a weight loss program because it helps tone and stimulate the gastro-intestinal system and reduces the gas that can be produced by a diet high in vegetables and fruits.

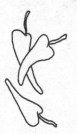

MY SECRET TO LOSING WEIGHT

The real secret to losing unwanted pounds and inches is to get the body to increase the amount of fuel it burns without sending it into panic anti-famine mode. To do this it needs a reasonable amount of many kinds of food and an adequate amount of exercise. Exercise need not be strenuous. I feel walking is one of the very best ways to exercise. Count your nutrients first. Then, calories tend to take care of themselves. And, when you eat healthy and move around a bit, your weight tends to take care of itself!

DANGER IN REDUCING CALORIES

Calorie restriction diets usually cause the loss of important muscle tissue as well as fat. The ratio can be significant. For many dieters, half of their weight loss is muscle or bone. Only half of it is the unwanted fat. Even with heavy exercise calorie restriction usually results in at least one-fourth of the weight coming from lean body mass.

To begin). Keep calories steady and increase movement.

It is important to eat some protein, as it is an important part of the system that tells your body when to stop eating. Some diets distort the value of protein by encouraging the dieter to eat huge amounts of it. These diets cause the body to

40

lose a lot of water, rapidly. This can make it seem as if there has been a sudden weight loss. Too much protein can increase the amount of precious calcium lost in the urinary tract and has been linked to more frequent bone fractures.

The healthiest way to eat protein is in proper proportion to other food. The protein space on my vinegar diet drawing shows you the proportion of protein the U.S. Department of Agriculture recommends in its Food Guide Pyramid.

WATER WASHES AWAY POUNDS

Water is especially important when losing weight. Drink at least eight full glasses a day. Coffee, tea and colas do not count as part of this. Extra water helps the body wash away toxins. It also encourages you to eat less. For variety, try water with a twist of lime, a wedge of lemon, a drop of vanilla or a dash of herbal vinegar. When you think you are really hungry it can help to drink a glass of water and wait a few minutes. You may find you are not so hungry after all!

VINEGAR IS ESSENTIAL

Vinegar, as acetic acid, is used by the body in the process by which it burns both carbohydrates and fat. It is naturally present in most plant and animal tissues. The human body even makes it. Vinegar also plays a role in how the body stores fat. When vinegar enters the blood stream it is carried to the kidneys and muscles. There, it either becomes energy or is used to make body tissues through its role in making essential amino acids. It even facilitates the process which forms the red blood cells that supply the body's oxygen!

FAST START TIPS

When you follow the vinegar weight loss plan for healthy eating your weight loss may not be sudden, but it will be permanent! You can give up yo-yo dieting that takes off a few pounds one week and puts them back on the next. The vinegar diet encourages you to eat a balanced diet, including food from all five food groups.

Bring out the good taste of these foods with healthy splashes of plain or flavored apple cider vinegar. It has only two calories in an entire tablespoon. Or, increase their nutrient content dramatically with fortified vinegars. If you follow this plan you will not have the overwhelming fatigue that goes with many diet plans. Actually, you should have more energy! Some other ways to get your weight loss program off to a fast start follow:

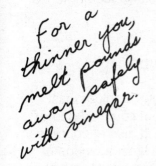

- Eat a raw vegetable or fruit half an hour before a meal.
- Eat only lean meats, and eat them less often.
- Add more cold water fish to your diet.
- Use small plates to serve your meals.
- Stop eating when you are full, even if food remains on your plate. You do not have to "clean up your plate."
- Substitute pureed pumpkin or apple sauce for half of the fat or oil in baked goods.
- Use only low fat dairy products.
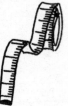
- Bake or simmer in no-fat sauces and broil rather than fry.
- Eat slowly because it takes about 20 minutes for the body to be able to judge when you are full.
- When you really want something you know is not good for you, eat at least one bite of it. In the long run you will be less likely to pig out on it!

VITAMINS & OTHER SUPPLEMENTS

Plants contain thousands of different substances. There is no way a pill can duplicate the exact effect of eating a fresh orange or a ripe tomato. The only way to get all the nutrients needed for a healthy body is to eat a variety of good foods. Regular exercise and enough pure water are also needed. This is a plan that is safe, sure and will bring results that last for life!

Many doctors recommend a daily vitamin and mineral supplement. This is partly because so many of the foods most people eat are so heavily processed. And, it is because so few people eat the five servings of fruits and vegetables recommended for good health.

As you make changes in your diet, do a little bit at a time. Use fats sparingly. Remember, all animal fats (and some vegetable fats) are associated with atherosclerosis. Do not shock your system with sudden changes in the way you eat or exercise. Strict calorie reduction can cause fatigue, and it makes the body's fat-burning mechanism slow down to conserve fuel. Even good things need to be done gradually!

Concentrate on high bulk, high fiber foods rather than concentrated sources of nutrients. Baked beans, for example, have lots of fiber, protein and are low fat. Mushrooms contain about 60 calories in an entire pound (25 calories in a cup). They are high in fiber and contain biotin, one of the complex of B vitamins involved in the digestion of fats and proteins. Some of the nutrients in mushrooms are only available to the body when they are cooked. Cooking also deactivates hydrazines in mushrooms that can increase the risk of getting cancer.

SPOT TONING

Yes, I believe you can reduce places on your body that are especially troublesome to you! Exercise which tones a particular set of muscles can give the appearance of spot reducing. For example, tummy toning can be achieved by increasing the strength of the abdominal muscles. These stronger muscles will hold a sagging tummy in and up, even if total fat mass stays the same. Strengthening back muscles can help you stand up straight and appear thinner, too.

Cream cheese is a fatty food!

FAT MAKES FAT!

If there is too much fat in your diet your body will use it instead of burning the body fat you want to lose. One way to use less fat is to substitute vinegar-based toppings for fatty sauces and spreads. It also helps to use butter or margarine at room temperature so you can spread it thinner. Apply it with a small spatula and you will use even less! Other ways to cut down on the fat in your diet follow:

Croissants + muffins are weighty food!

FATTY FOOD	BETTER CHOICE
Sour cream	Whipped cottage cheese
Cheese omelette	Egg substitute scrambled with vegetables
Granola	Oatmeal with raisins
Beef & cheese nachos	Bean burrito
Fettuccine Alfredo	Spaghetti with tomato sauce
Sweet & sour pork	Pork stir fry
Hamburger, fries, milk shake	Salad, baked potato, tea
Loaded pizza	Vegetarian pizza
Packaged microwave popcorn	Air-popped popcorn
Danish	Fruit
Whole milk	Skim milk
Deep fried chicken leg	Broiled, skinless chicken breast

LOSE A LITTLE, GAIN A LOT!

Why lose weight? Because even a small weight loss can give you a lot of benefits. Diabetes, high blood pressure, atherosclerosis, heart disease and cancer are all tied to extra body fat. Even a little weight off can decrease risk of osteoarthritis, even in your hands. (Researchers think a chemical in stored fat increases the progression of osteoarthritis.)

Where and when you gain matters, too. Extra pounds on your stomach are more serious than weight carried on the hips and thighs. And, if you have gained more than 10 pounds since becoming an adult it is more of a problem than if you have always carried the extra weight. This "middle-of-life" weight gain is especially dangerous for women. A mere 10 pounds can raise the risk of heart attack by 25%. (25 pounds may triple it!) Gaining weight as an adult tends to increase blood fat, pressure and sugar levels.

You can lose weight with no drugs or harmful side effects.

VISUALIZATION

Put your daydreams to work for you and they will become reality! You can use visualization to reshape your body. It makes any weight reduction program more effective. Some say you can even increase your metabolism this way. Put a picture in your mind of your new thin self. Enjoy the way it will feel. Do this before you get out of bed in the morning, during meals, and as you drop off to sleep at night. Soon it will be real.

AROMATHERAPY

Smell is 90% of the body's sensation of taste. Researchers are using this to help people lose weight. They have found that, for some people, smelling banana, peppermint or apple allows them to keep from overeating. Average weight loss using aromatherapy is about a pound a week. These smells probably work by making the body think it has eaten. Fennel may also be an appetite suppressant.

VARIETY! VARIETY!

We know the body needs a variety of smells and tastes at each meal to satisfy its food cravings. Be sure to include sweet and sour, salty and tangy foods in your diet, along with a range of colors.

Experiment with new and different foods at the supermarket. Try a pre-made salad, tiny baby carrots or a prepared selection of vegetables such as broccoli and cauliflower. They may be more expensive than your usual way of buying vegetables, but compared to eating out or a packaged "diet food" meal they are cheap. Their wonderful nutritional benefits are worth it if this is the only way you are going to eat these healthy foods.

THE FRENCH CONNECTION

Wine and France have an inescapable connection. It is home of some of the great wines of the world. And wine is one of the substances from which an excellent vinegar is made. Wine, like vinegar, is an acidic liquid, much like the chemistry of the body. It has long been recognized as an aid to digestion. Now it is said to do even more!

Many believe a small glass of wine with or before meals can have a definite effect on weight. It does this because it seems to reduce the total amount of fuel the body desires. The effect is especially noticeable when compared to the effect of unsweetened liquids.

Red grapes, from which red wine vinegar is made, have been found to contain a very special antioxidant. This substance, proanthocyanidin, is extremely effective at fighting free radicals associated with degenerative diseases and aging.

FASTING — IS IT FOR YOU?

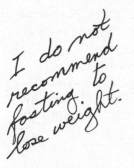

A weight-loss fast is a period of time where only liquids are taken. It can bring about an immediate small amount of weight loss, but because it throws the body into famine protection mode it is of very limited long term value. Weight lost through fasting inevitably returns, often within a day or two. It is not a way to permanently lose weight.

Arthritis sufferers sometimes use a fast to control pain. It has been found that fasting changes immune cells, so some kinds of arthritis may be calmed by a fast. Although fasting may bring temporary relief, it must not be overused. A low fat and protein diet that has lots of vegetables and fruits may work just as well.

If you decide to fast while on the vinegar weight loss diet be sure to supplement the vinegar and honey tonic with large amounts of vegetable and fruit juices. And, keep the fast short. Prolonged fasting can cause serious damage to the body!

ET SAYS   IS THE VINEGAR WEIGHT LOSS DIET FOR YOU?

Ask your doctor before beginning any changes to your usual diet! Feel free to show your health care provider the drawings that show you how to fill your plate for the vinegar weight loss diet. And please remember — suggestions offered in the vinegar diet may be appropriate for healthy adults — they are not intended for children, the frail elderly, those taking medications or with chronic health conditions — without the approval of a medical professional!

Chapter Five

Build Up Your Body with Vinegar

The vinegar diet can help you create the stronger body you have always wanted! With its help I feel you can gain strength, energy and vigor.

Many older adults, particularly those who live alone, are at risk for becoming too thin. If body weight is too low the immune system may not be getting all the nutrients it needs to keep the body healthy. Frequent colds and bouts of flu, having several allergies, slow healing of cuts and scrapes and being tired every day could mean you have a weak immune system. Because very low body weight can lead to greater susceptibility to disease, if you are thin it is extra-important to eat some food, each day, from each food group.

My vinegar diet can be a healthy beginning for building up a frail, too thin, undermuscled or flabby body. If you are underweight or disabled, you – most of all – need the nutrients of vegetables, fruits and whole grains. Use the drawing in Chapter Three every time you eat. It shows you how much of each food group to eat at each meal.

It is essential to use these proportions every time you eat! THE SECRET TO BUILDING UP YOUR BODY WITH THE VINEGAR DIET IS PROPORTION!! Every day, you need to include foods in your diet from all five food groups.

Add healthy oils for extra calories and smooth taste, fortified vinegars for concentrated nutrients, a few sweets, and drink six to eight glasses of water a day. To maintain an average weight and to get the nutrients your body needs each day, you need:

• 6 to 11 servings of breads and grains
• 3 to 5 servings of vegetables
• 2 to 4 servings of fruits

- 2 to 3 servings of protein
- 2 to 3 servings of dairy products
- Enough oil or fats to maintain weight
- A bit of sugar or sweets

To build up your body, choose foods with concentrated calories and nutrients. Eat bananas instead of grapes, avocados rather than watermelon, corn or beets rather than lettuce or mushrooms. All beans are good for you because they are rich sources of the protein you need to build up a damaged or frail body. You may tolerate small meals every three hours better than three large meals.

FATS

Fats are the most concentrated fuel for your body, as well as being an essential part of the taste, flavor and texture of food. For the same bulk, fat has more than twice the calories of other food. Because saturated fats, such as those from meats, may be associated with a higher risk of clogged arteries, choose healthy vegetable oils. Hazelnut, walnut and flaxseed oils are good choices for mixing with vinegars. So are monounsaturated corn, safflower and soy oils. For cooking, use oils that are resistant to heat, such as canola or olive.

fat has 9 calories per gram, protein and carbo-hydrates have 4.

EXERCISE

Exercise is as important for normalizing weight as diet! It increases energy and lifts your mood. Your first goal should be to increase endurance and flexibility. To begin, stand up straight and breath deeply. Get oxygen flowing to all parts of your body. Short walks throughout the day help do this.

Regular, gentle exercise will increase the body's ability to move and bend and firm up flabby muscles. Begin by doing several repeats of light exercises, rather than trying to do heavy exercises too soon. Twenty minutes of exercise, three times a week can add years to your life. It is not necessary to do all 20 minutes at once. It is often better to start out exercising a few minutes at a time, spread out during the day.

48

When physical problems slow you down exercise may seem like the last thing you need to do. Actually, it is probably more important for those with physical problems to exercise than for others. Move the parts of the body that you can. If you use a walker or cane, you still need to move your body as much as possible to retain balance and coordination. Do a lot of stretching and range of motion exercises to keep joints mobile.

Exercise is needed for bones to retain their calcium. Only a small part of the body's total calcium circulates in the blood, so tests can show a blood level that is normal, even when the bones are honeycombed by loss of calcium.

Mild exercise is especially important for those with fibromyalgia or any other type of arthritis. Gentle exercise is needed to strengthen tendons and ligaments around joints. Those with mild high blood pressure may find exercise lowers it into normal range.

IS THE BEST WAY TO FITNESS TOO EASY?

The President's Council on Physical Fitness and Sports calls walking the slower, surer way to fitness! Walking burns about the same number of calories as running, for the same distance. The best news of all is that the less you weigh, the fewer calories you burn and the more you weigh, the more calories you burn in this easiest of exercises. Many researchers believe walking is better than running for overall body conditioning. Generally, those who walk regularly even sleep better.

For best results swing your arms while you walk. It is also a good idea to do stretching exercises at the beginning and end of your walk. Take it slowly at first. If walking makes you too breathless to talk, you are going too fast.
Getting some exercise is more important than how fast you go or how far. The biggest benefits come when those who do not usually exercise begin moving. Advantages to walking for exercise include:

- No lessons are needed, almost everyone can do it without training.
- You can do it most any time, anywhere.
- It is free.
- No special equipment is needed.

Expensive "sports drinks" are unnecessary. A teaspoon each of vinegar and honey stirred into a quart of water makes a good substitute. Or, plain water will do fine!

Exercise tends to normalize appetite. The body goes on burning more fuel for hours after exercise. Firm, healthy muscles burn more fuel, even at rest, than soft, flabby fat. Exercise and the extra nutrition of fortified vinegar can aid in lowering cholesterol, boost the immune system, restore age-wasted muscles and more.

FATIGUE

Chronic fatigue is not a natural part of aging. It is a sign something is wrong, perhaps that the immune system is not functioning at its peak level. To find out why you are overly tired, decide when it happens most. When are you exhausted? Keep a chart for a week and write down the time you are really tired each day. Then, look back and see how this relates to your eating habits.

 Be especially aware of your use of caffeine, too. It may increase fatigue symptoms. Low levels of the B complex of vitamins reduces endurance and results in feelings of tiredness. Using music to help energize your body and lift your mood may also help.

You may need to add a protein, carbohydrate and calcium rich snack for an afternoon energy boost. Cheese and crackers, with a rich honey and strawberry fortified vinegar to dip them in tastes great. Or, try a slice of chicken on half an English muffin and a spoonful of cooked prunes drizzled with cucumber-celery fortified vinegar. Wash it down with skim milk. A short afternoon nap may help, too.

If you are very thin, use the principals of thermogenesis and help the body conserve heat. Be sure to wear a heavy sweater when it is cool so the body does not need to burn a lot of calories to stay warm.

Fight fatigue by eating healthy food, getting daily exercise and taking an active interest in the world around you. My goal is to help you stay fit so you can manage your daily life.

Chapter Six

Recipes For Success

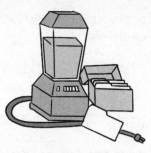

If weight is a problem, you need a better way of eating, not another "diet!" We have come a long way from the days when it was thought food left on the table overnight fed the fairies, thus ensuring good fortune for the household. We now know it is the cook who shapes the fortunes of the household by preparing healthy food!

Hundreds of foods make use of the preservative and unique taste qualities of vinegar. It is an essential ingredient in catsup and mayonnaise, and is one of the original preservatives for meats and eggs. The rich, vivid taste sensation of fortified vinegar can help stimulate an appetite which has become dulled with age or depression.

Vegetables have fiber, vitamins and minerals. They are low in salt and most are fat-free. Beta-carotene rich vegetables fight colon, lung, bladder and esophagus cancer. A special carotenoid (lutein) fights deterioration of the retina. All foods with soluble fiber, such as the apples used to make apple cider vinegar, are good for preventing heart disease. A few recipes for using vinegar in a healthy diet follow:

EASY YOGURT To 1/2 gallon skim milk add 1 tablespoon each apple cider vinegar and plain, live culture yogurt. Mix every well, cap lightly, and set in a warm place for about 24 hours. Drain off excess clear liquid and you have a mild yogurt. Or, shake the mixture for a cultured buttermilk drink. This is a great way to use milk that is a bit old.

NO-FAT COLE SLAW Sprinkle 1/4 cup sugar over 4 cups shredded cabbage. Let set overnight. Add 2 cups cucumber-celery fortified vinegar and mix well.

HOT ORANGE BEETS Simmer 1/2 cup champagne vinegar, 1/2 cup beet juice and 1 teaspoon cayenne pepper until reduced by half. Add 4 cups canned, sliced beets and 2 cups chopped fresh orange. Simmer until just warm and top with 1 teaspoon parsley. Serve warm or chill overnight.

PEACHY FISH Baste fish fillets with fortified peach vinegar and bake or broil until well done.

CUCUMBER BOATS Cut a cucumber lengthwise and scoop out the seeds. Fill with a mixture made of equal parts fortified vinegar, yogurt, diced tomatoes and celery.

VINEGAR SUNDAE Top your favorite ice cream with a fortified fruit vinegar for a super-delicious sundae. Thick, fruity vinegars make an interesting change for topping pancakes or French toast, too.

RASPBERRY SLIPPER Put 1 tablespoon fortified raspberry vinegar in a tall glass and fill with cold water. This is a good way to get your daily vinegar and add water to your diet. This bit of sweetness before mealtime helps control the appetite and is just plain good!

TANGY CHERRIES Steep pitted sweet cherries for 3 hours in enough wine to barely cover them. Then add enough champagne vinegar to double the volume and simmer, uncovered for 15 minutes. Remove from heat and top with generous dashes of hot pepper and cinnamon. Add honey if a sweeter mixture is desired.

SALADS

Top salads with a dressing made of vegetable stock and vinegar instead of using oil. For a fat-free stock simmer a mix of diced summer vegetables in lots of water. When they are tender, puree the mix in a blender. For a darker, more intense stock, brown vegetables before simmering. Use herbal vinegars for variety, fortified vinegars for bolder flavors and extra nutrients.

PASTA & TUNA SALAD Toss together a can of well-drained tuna, 1 cup diced celery, 2 cups cooked pasta, 1 cup halved seedless red grapes, 1/2 cup white raisins, 1 cup diced, unpeeled apples. For the dressing, use 1/4 cup yogurt mixed with the liquid from the tuna.

FULL MEAL SALAD Combine 1 cup each of the following cooked

vegetables: green, yellow wax, pinto and lima beans. Add 1 cup each chick peas, green peas and diced potatoes. Mix in 1/2 cup onion and 1/4 cup parsley. Toss with vinegar blended half and half with liquid from cooking the vegetables.

POTATO-CARROT SALAD Mix 2 cups boiled, diced potatoes and carrots. Toss with a dressing made of 1/4 cup apple cider vinegar, 1/4 cup tomato paste, 1 teaspoon chili powder, 1 tablespoon parsley.

CITRUS SALAD Peel and chop 1 cup oranges and 1 cup grapefruit. Top with raspberry, blueberry or strawberry fortified vinegar.

RECIPE TIPS

Get meals off to a healthy start with homemade soup. Good choices include chicken, celery, pumpkin and vegetable. In clear soups, use the liquid from canned vegetables or the water used to cook fresh ones. It can contain nearly one-third of the total nutrients. Pep up mild chicken soup with a splash of herbal vinegar or a bit of fortified garlic vinegar. Rinse cooked meats for soups (such as hamburger) in water to remove their fat. Prepare healthy cream soups by using skim milk made with twice the normal milk powder.

Use mustard, ketchup or apple butter on breads and rolls instead of fatty spreads. Better yet, drizzle them with fortified vinegar or cottage cheese blended with apple cider vinegar.

Cook stuffing outside a chicken or turkey to avoid the risk of salmonella germs. As a bonus, it will be lower in calories than the exact same stuffing cooked inside fowl! (If cooked in the bird, stuffing soaks up melted fat.) For a healthy change try white or brown rice instead of bread for stuffing. Use tomatoes, corn, mushrooms and red and green peppers, too.

Skip the salt in boiling pasta and vegetables. Substitute a splash of apple cider or herbal vinegar.

Make lighter corn muffins and brownies by replacing half the oil with apple sauce, mashed pumpkin or sweet potato.

An easy, tasty dessert can be made by baking bananas, pears or apples with cinnamon and nutmeg.

Add a bit of peppermint to salads for a fresh taste. It is said to sharpen the memory and stimulate circulation.

Skim milk tastes better with a tablespoon or so of dry milk stirred into each glass. A dash of vanilla or honey makes it even better. Add dry skim milk to mashed potatoes, cooked cereal, gravy, ground meats, casseroles, and baked goods to increase the amount of calcium you eat. Be sure to finish the milk at the bottom of the cereal bowl because many nutrients dissolve into it. For a fruity milk treat mix 3/4 cup very cold skim milk, 1/4 cup frozen orange juice concentrate and 1/4 cup crushed ice.

FOOD FACTS

Olive oil is graded by flavor as extra virgin, virgin and fine. There is no difference in calories. Canola oil has linolenic acid, an omega-3 fatty acid (usually found in cold water fish) for a healthy heart.

One green pepper has much more vitamin C than a large orange. When peppers fully mature and turn red, their beta carotene content increases dramatically.

Sweet potatoes and white potatoes have a similar number of calories, sweet ones have lots of vitamin C and beta carotene.

Avocados contain more fat than other vegetables. Dry roasted nuts have most of the calories of regular roasted nuts.

Spinach and other flavored pastas are not good sources of vegetable nutrients. There are just enough vegetables added to make them have interesting colors. Usually this is a tablespoon or less in an entire pound of pasta!

FOOD CAUTIONS

Some foods need to be used with caution. Tofu can develop a bacteria that causes gastrointestinal distress if it is not stored in the refrigerator.

Limit the amount of liver you eat because it collects and stores any toxins the animal may have eaten.

Salmonella contamination is becoming very frequent in meat and eggs. E. coli (Escherichia coli) can be found in meats, milk and juices which have not been pasteurized. For best health, never eat raw meat, fish or eggs. This includes cookie dough, uncooked eggnog and cake batter. Disinfect utensils used on these foods by soaking them in white vinegar. And, keep cold foods cold, hot foods hot.

Chapter Seven

Ageless Beauty & Glowing Skin

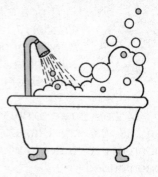

The vinegar diet does more than energize the inside of the body. This healthy regime will help the outside of the body look its very best. Your increased energy level will give your skin the glow of fresh health because when you are good to your insides, your outsides will show it!

For hundreds of years vinegar has been the basis for home remedies to beautify, cleanse and soothe the skin. Some of the most helpful ways that have been suggested, through the years, for using vinegar follow:

SOOTHING BATHS

Add a generous splash of apple cider vinegar to bath water to help keep the skin soft and smooth. Vinegar helps soothe itchy skin, while discouraging germs. Make bath time super-special by using an herbal scented vinegar. Especially nice vinegars for the tub include rose, lilac, geranium, lavender, rosemary, thyme and mint. (Some scented vinegars are only appropriate for external use.)

A few tablespoons of honey added to apple cider vinegar in a tub of warm bath water helps moisturize skin.

FACIALS

Blend together 1/2 cup apple cider vinegar and 1/4 cup well-cooked rice and 1/4 cup cooked oatmeal. Spread this mixture on the face, neck and shoulders. Allow to dry for 10 minutes, then wash off and pat dry with a soft towel. Skin will be soft and smooth.

For a refining facial, combine 1 tablespoon apple cider vinegar, 1 tablespoon honey and 1/2 a mashed banana. Apply a generous coating and after five minutes your skin will feel revitalized. Strawberries or a peach may be used in place of the banana.

Make a paste of dry yeast and warm water. Pat this onto the face and allow to dry. Rinse off with warm water. Then, rinse again with a quart of cool water to which a tablespoon of apple cider vinegar has been added.

HANDS & FEET

Thoroughly blend 1/2 cup olive oil and 1 cup mashed potatoes. It should have a cream-like consistency. Rub this mixture onto hands and feet to smooth and moisturize rough skin.

Eating lots of cauliflower fortified vinegar will give the body extra amounts of biotin. This plant-based nutrient helps it grow strong nails.

Clean and soothe work roughened hands with a paste of apple cider vinegar and cornmeal. After a minute or two rinse with warm water and apply a soothing lotion.

For silky feeling hands, wet them with apple cider vinegar. Then, rub them very gently with sugar. When the sugar is dissolved rinse hands in warm water. They will feel extraordinarily soft and velvety.

Condition hands and feet by soaking them for 15 minutes in 1 cup cooked oatmeal, 1/2 cup milk and 1/2 cup apple cider vinegar.

Banish foot odor by soaking feet in strong tea. Follow with a rinse made from 1 cup warm water and 1 cup apple cider vinegar.

Vinegar has been used to control more than foot odor. It was once considered an underarm deodorant! And, vinegar has been used as a gargle to deal with unpleasant breath. Herbal vinegars are said to be especially helpful. Vinegars which are especially good breath fresheners include rosemary, sage, clove, thyme, cinnamon and any of the mints. Because too much exposure to vinegar can hurt tooth enamel, always rinse with clear water after using it in the mouth.

SUNBURN, CANCER & CAROTENOIDS

Carotenoids, those amazing substances in vegetables and fruits, can reduce sunburn damage by UV rays! New research indicates eating carotenoid rich vegetables and fruits can be a preventive against skin cancer. It has been suggested that supplements of carotenoids, taken before going out in the sun, may be as effective as sun screens. This is another reason to use fortified vinegars to increase the amount of these foods in your diet!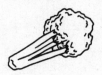

Chapter Eight

Vinegar & Disease

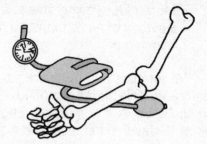

An ancient proverb assures us "Diet cures more than doctors." Combine this age-old wisdom with the importance of vinegar and you have — the vinegar diet!

My vinegar diet brings together the goodness of vinegar and eating habits needed for continuing health. I believe the balance of food in the vinegar diet furnishes your body with what it needs to resist disease and be vital and vigorous well into old age.

THE VINEGAR DIET IS SOUND NUTRITION FOR A HEALTHY HEART!

Basics of the vinegar diet have been followed by health conscious individuals for decades. What is new, is scientific confirmation that there is a direct association between food and specific diseases. Substances in foods are now linked with arthritis and rheumatism, asthma, allergies, colds and flu, Alzheimer's Disease, diabetes, blood pressure, cancer, heart and cardiovascular disease. Improper eating habits can lead to a depressed immune system and even to more rapid aging!

Twenty-five national health and aging organizations, including the American Dietetic Association, National Council on the Aging and American Academy of Family Physicians issued a report on Medical Nutrition Therapy. They propose using foods as medical treatment because many elders' eating habits put them at risk for malnutrition. They suggest preventive health care in the form of nutritional intervention would result in an older population with better immune function, resulting in:

• Fewer medical complications.
• Shorter hospital stays.

- More elders being able to live independently, in their own homes.
- Savings of more than 100 million dollars a year in medical expenses.

Vegetables and fruits are storehouses of antioxidants such as beta carotene. This wondrous antioxidant has the ability to neutralize free radicals. So, it is no surprise degenerative diseases of aging are less likely to develop in those with high blood levels of the more than 50 carotenoids in vegetables and fruits.

Anti-oxidants in vegetables & fruits attack free radicals.

Each carotenoid seems to protect a particular part of the body or type of cell. They also have different ways of providing this antioxidant protection. Some foods, and what they contain follow:

Cantaloupe, carrots & pumpkin — alpha carotene.
Apricots, carrots, pumpkin & sweet potatoes — beta carotene.
Oranges, peaches & tangerines — beta cryptoxanthin.
Apricots & tomatoes — gamma carotene.
Red peppers, mustard greens & corn — lutein.
Tomatoes & watermelon — lycopene.
Beet tops & kale — zeaxanthin.

ILLNESS & DIET

General aging of the brain has been linked to damage caused by free radicals. Specifically, confusion and memory loss can be caused by too little vitamin B-12 or folic acid. Some depression is associated with a deficiency of folic acid, calcium, iron, copper, magnesium or potassium. Protect the mind from aging and depression by eating a diet high in antioxidant containing fruits and vegetables!

Macular degeneration is fought by the lutein and zeaxanthin in kale, spinach and several kinds of peppers.

Dark green and orange vegetables are rich in carotenoids that the body converts to vitamin A. It is needed by the body to make rhodopsin. This substance is essential to night vision and helps cut the risk of developing macular degeneration, one of the most common causes of blindness.

Prostate, breast and endometrial cancers seem to be restrained by lycopene. It is a carotenoid in tomatoes, pink grapefruit, apricots and watermelon.

Calcium loss from bones and menopause symptoms can both be reduced by estrogen-like isoflavones in soybeans.

Psoriasis is less common in those who eat lots of fresh fruit, carrots and tomatoes.

Urinary tract infections are inhibited by phytocompounds in blueberries and cranberries.

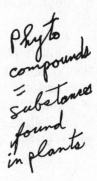

Phyto compounds = substances found in plants

ARTHRITIS, ALLERGIES & MORE

Food allergies can cause a feeling of extreme fatigue after meals. Foods can also cause bloating, congestion, itching, cramping, headaches and mood swings. Food sensitivity, a less dramatic reaction, has been linked to fatigue and joint pain.

The existence of allergic arthritis shows how very much food affects the immune system. Researchers are constantly adding to the medical community's knowledge of how food allergies can cause the body to produce chemicals that trigger inflammatory reactions.

Those with arthritis may be particularly susceptible to food reactions because their immune systems already react in inappropriate ways. Zinc, magnesium, copper, vitamin B-6 and folic acid help regulate the immune system and may also minimize the side effects of anti-arthritis drugs.

Many seasonings do more than make foods taste better. Arthritis pain may sometimes be eased by the actions of cayenne, ginger or turmeric. (No, hot foods such as cayenne peppers do not cause ulcers.)

Foods affect the bacteria naturally present in the digestive system. Some have been linked to making rheumatoid arthritis symptoms worse.

Mushrooms contain polysaccharides, complex carbohydrates

that stimulate the body's natural immune response to both bacteria and viruses. They have been used for thousands of years in Eastern medicine to fight disease.

Doctors are searching for better ways to fight deadly infections, such as tuberculosis, with diet changes. I believe that one day they will confirm the existence of specific foods that have the ability to regulate the immune system. In the meantime, most recommend a low saturated fat regimen that features lots of vegetables and fruits and a minimum of animal protein.

Alfalfa has been proved to induce systemic lupus erythematosus. This inflammatory disease of the connective tissue can flare up after eating large quantities of alfalfa sprouts, seeds or tablets. And, those who already have lupus, but are in a remission, can reactivate the disease by eating alfalfa. Researchers suspect a non-protein amino acid in alfalfa (L-canavanine) may cause blood changes in those predisposed to lupus.

UN - CLOGGING ARTERIES

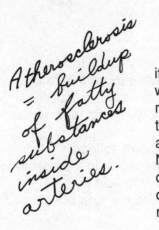

Atherosclerosis = buildup of fatty substances inside arteries.

"Coronary artery disease can be stopped in its tracks, even reversed, without drugs!" That is what researchers say about an eating plan very much like the vinegar diet. Their studies suggest the nutrients found in abundance in vegetables and fruits can improve the condition of arteries. Nutrition therapy can help even if there are no obvious signs of deficiencies. Extra amounts of vitamin C, chromium, magnesium, selenium, niacin and potassium are especially helpful.

New studies report those who eat a salad every day have fewer heart attacks. When eggplant is eaten with foods high in vitamin C it seems to protect the body from developing fatty plaques in the arteries. Vegetables are excellent foods, but they do not take the place of fruits. Eating both fresh fruits and vegetables, every day, has been linked to a significant reduction in fatal heart attacks and strokes.

Ginger is very good for artery health. It helps lower cholesterol and seems to discourage cells from sticking together to form clots.

FIBER

A low fat, high fiber diet helps deter heart attacks, strokes and cancer. One way fiber fights cancer is by quickly pushing toxin laden food through the colon. Fiber helps reduce the likelihood of developing stomach ulcers because food and its digestive acids spend less time in the body. Its bulk eases constipation and its water absorbing capabilities moderates diarrhea.

Soluble fiber in legumes such as pinto, navy, kidney and soy beans protects good HDL cholesterol and lowers bad LDL. They begin their cholesterol lowering work almost immediately.

Fiber, particularly the soluble fiber in foods like oatmeal, helps remove cholesterol from the body. Too much fiber, such as is in some supplements can interfere with calcium absorption.

The membrane holding together sections of grapefruit is an especially healthy fiber. Half of it is soluble to soak up cholesterol, half is insoluble to fight constipation and colon cancer. Two grapefruit have a full day's fiber needs.

Vinegars fortified with apples or sweet potatoes are high fiber foods that can help ease hemorrhoids.

Diabetes is at least as deadly for adult women as breast cancer! A high fiber, low fat, diet and exercise are the recommended preventatives.

CANCER

More than half of women's cancers can be traced to diet. Breasts seem to be particularly sensitive to food toxins such as pesticides and partially hydrogenated oil preservatives. This is probably because these oil soluble chemicals tend to be stored in breast fat.

Lower the risk of breast cancer by eating soy products for their phytoestrogens (plant estrogens). Eat broccoli, cauliflower and kale for their effect on the way the body uses estrogen.

Increase fiber SLOWLY to prevent cramps & gas.

Garlic is considered an anti-cancer food because it stops the activity of some substances which are known to cause cancer. It seems to work on both existing cancers and as a preventive against new ones. Garlic lowers the risk of developing many diseases because it strengthens the immune system.

FAT

All fuels produce by-products when they are burned. Some of these by-products are more harmful than others. Foods high in saturated fats produce more toxic chemicals than vegetables, fruits and whole grains. Some fat is necessary for good health, even the body makes a bit of cholesterol.

The healthiest diet seems to be one with a small amount of the right kinds of oil added to it.

Polyunsaturated oils such as flaxseed, corn, safflower and soy are good for use in cold dishes. Flaxseed is a rich source of the omega-3 oils also found in cold water fish.

When polyunsaturated oils are heated they produce toxic lipid peroxides. So, for cooking, the oleic acid containing monounsaturated oils are best. Two good heat and light resistant monounsaturated oils are olive and canola.

Fat substitutes are used in many processed foods. Simplesse is one that has been used for many years. Avicel is a cellulose gel. N-Oil is a tapioca based dextrin. Olestra, one of the newest fat substitutes, is calorie free, but may inhibit fat soluble vitamins such as A, D, E and K. It may also interfere with the absorption of important carotenoids.

WEIGHT LOSS DRUGS

Weight loss drugs work in several ways. Some of the newest ones affect the way serotonin, a neurotransmitter, is handled by the brain. This is thought to be helpful for some people because neurotransmitters affect the way the body's appetite control mechanism works. A few weight loss drugs that are available now, or are being tested, and some things you need to know about them, follow:

REDUX is the trade name for dexfenfluramine. It raises brain levels of serotonin and so produces results similar to anti-depression drugs such as Prozac. Redux can complicate the condition of those with high blood pressure. Its manufacturer recently sent letters to 300,000 health care providers to warn of newly documented side effects, including primary pulmonary hypertension, a potentially deadly reaction.

PONDIMIN is a trade name for fenfluramine. IONAMIN and FASTIN are trade names for phentermine. These drugs are not recommended for anyone taking blood pressure lowering agents, antidepressants, or anyone who has a history of alcohol or drug abuse. Their side effects can include insomnia, headache, diarrhea and nausea.

Fen-Phen is the popular name for the combination of fenfluramine and phentermine, two appetite suppressing drugs.

Drugs being tested include orlistat, sibutramine and leptin, a hormone found in fat cells. Researchers have been working with leptin for more than 10 years in the hope of developing an obesity fighting drug. It still seems linked to insomnia, constipation and increased blood pressure. And, patients tend to regain lost weight when it is discontinued.

Some widely publicized drugs for weight loss have had problems with the Federal Drug Administration (FDA). Some injections of adrenal cortex extract have been linked to serious bacterial infections. They are the subject of a Federal Drug Administration alert. The FDA has tried to ban the use of Co-enzyme Q-10, a substance that is associated with the body's regulation of metabolism.

The FDA warns that those who take many of the prescription appetite suppressants increase their risk of developing primary pulmonary hypertension by as much as 20 times. Diarrhea, dizziness, memory lapses and depression are common short-term side effects of weight loss drugs. Long-term studies on safety and effectiveness have not yet been completed.

Experts agree, when dieters stop taking drugs most can expect to gain back the weight which was lost. They are then faced with the need to take the drugs on and off for the rest of their lives. (Plus the cost of repeated doctor visits and about $50.00 a month for the pills.) For most people the risks "out weigh" any weight problem!

A nonprescription supplement, chromium picolinate, seems to have fewer known side effects than some other weight loss agents. But there have been no long term tests to confirm this. And, it has not been proven effective for most people.

Caffeine is the most popular stimulant drug in the world! Until 1991 caffeine was used in over-the-counter weight loss products. The FDA no longer permits this, as it has been deemed to have no long term effect on weight. Colas, regular tea, coffee and chocolate contain caffeine.

Caffeine increases metabolism, especially when combined with aspirin. Unfortunately it also encourages brittle bones. It is estimated that one six ounce cup of coffee pulls about five milligrams of calcium from the body. Replacing this calcium takes the equivalent of the concentrated power of two tablespoons of yogurt.

Cafestol and kahweol are in the oils in ground coffee. They are not in instant or filtered drip coffee, but remain in percolated coffee. Drinking even four cups a day of oil-containing coffee may significantly increase the risk of heart disease.

One thing all weight loss drugs share is that when they are stopped, any weight lost tends to be regained! Considering their many, often dangerous, side effects they are a poor substitute for a healthy diet and a little exercise.

FOOD & CHEMO-PREVENTIVES

Turmeric is a very safe, anti-UV radiation, antioxidant. It has even been shown to help prevent chromosome damage.

Rosemary contains substances that act against free radicals. It also protects the liver from the damage that can be done by some toxins. Rosemary's phenolic compounds, carnosol and carnosic acid do this antioxidant work. These flavonoids can be used as preservatives for fats in foods.

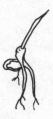

Ginger has substances to help protect the liver. It is also useful against platelet clumping, which contributes to heart attacks.

Apples, onions and tea contain flavonoids, antioxidants to reduce the risk of heart disease.

Carotenoids, those amazing substances in vegetables and fruits, can help limit the spread of breast cancer. Tests are being conducted on using them to stop the spread of lung, stomach and colon cancers, too.

Beta carotene helps maintain healthy eyes. When taken at the same time as aspirin, it may prevent some side effects, such as stomach distress.

Garlic has substances that energize the immune system. One of these, selenium, has been found to lower the risk of cancer of the colon, lung, prostate and rectum.

All weight loss drugs carry some health warnings. Vegetables, fruits and whole grains do not. Whenever a product has dangers attached to it, proceed with great caution. You may not need to take that risk. The vinegar diet, with its use of fortified vinegars to add all the goodness of vegetables and fruits to your diet may be what you need.

No matter what scientists finally decide about vinegar's usefulness in the diet, people have instinctively felt, for untold centuries, that vinegar was good for them. It is truly a living substance, capable of bringing health benefits far beyond the ability of today's medical world to fully comprehend!

Chapter Nine

Questions & Answers

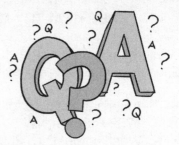

Question: I have diabetes, a heart condition, arthritis, etc. Is it safe for me to take vinegar every day?

Answer: If you have a chronic medical condition ALWAYS check with a health care professional before adding anything, including vinegar, to your diet.

Question: I take medication. Can vinegar be taken with it?

Answer: If you take medication, including over the counter drugs, ALWAYS check with a health care professional before adding vinegar to your diet.

Question: Will vinegar pull calcium from my bones?

Answer: No. Vinegar in the digestive system does not come into direct contact with your bones. It works in other ways to aid health.

Question: What kind of vinegar should I use?

Answer: Use white vinegar for cleaning and to pickle light colored foods. Use apple cider vinegar for tonics and most recipes. Rice, champagne, wine and other vinegars can also be used in recipes.

Question: Where can I find herbal vinegars?

Answer: More and more supermarkets now carry a line of herbal vinegars. For the freshest, most robust flavor make your own by adding a few tablespoons of an herb to a good supermarket vinegar.

Question: Where can I find organic vinegar?

Answer: A few supermarkets now carry organic vinegar, as do many health food stores. Some mail order speciality houses sell organic vinegar, too.

FREE HEALTHY-EATING PUBLICATIONS

For information on how the chemicals in plants (phytochemicals) fight disease send a stamped, self addressed, business sized envelope to:

American Institute for Cancer Research
1759 R Street NW
Washington, D.C. 20009

YOU CAN HELP DOCUMENT THE EFFECTS OF THE VINEGAR DIET!

Would you like to add your experiences to my register of vinegar diet results? Simply follow the guidelines in Chapter Three, Four or Five for at least three months. Be sure to eat lots of fruits, vegetables and grains, limit fats and sweets, and begin a walking or other program of gentle exercise.

Then write and let me know how the diet affected you. I want to know if it helped you move your weight into a healthier range. Be sure to tell me exactly how much difference my vinegar diet made to your weight and to your general health. If you shared the plate drawing with your doctor, tell me what reaction you received. Send your vinegar diet results to:

Diet Survey
% Emily Thacker
PO Box 980
Hartville, OH 44632

REFERENCES

"Action Almanac" UFCW Action. March- April 1993: p 14

ALIAS C. and Linden G. "Food Biochemistry." Professors of Biochemistry, University of Nancy, France: Ellis Harwood Series in Food Science and Technology: 1991.

AMELLAL, M. et al. "Inhibition of Mast Cell Histamine Release by Flavonoids and Bioflavonoids," Planta Medica. Stuttgart: Georg Thieme Verlag, vol 49, 1985: pp 16-19.

AMERICAN Heart Association, "Brand Name Fat and Cholesterol Counter." Bristol-Myers Squibb Co. NY, NY: Times Books, 1994.

ANDERSON- Parrado, Patricia; "No Mater How You Slice 'Tomato' You'll Get Lycopene in Every Bite." Better Nutrition Dec. 1996: p 14.
"An Interview With Durk Pearson and Sandy Shaw:" pp 1-5

ANTOL, Marie Nadine. "Healing Teas" Garden City Park, NY: Avery Publishing Group;1996.
"Arthritis Update." Nov-Dec 1996, vol III/no 6

BOWERS, Jane. "Food Theory and Applications." NY, NY: Macmillan Publishing Co. 1992.

BRODY, Jane E. "Midlife Weight Gain is Very Dangerous to Your Health." Health Confidential, vol 9/ no 5: p. 5.

CARPER, Jean "Food-Your Miracle Medicine." NY NY: Harper Collins Publishers, 1993.

CHAITOW, Leon. "Amino Acids in Therapy." Northamptonshire, England: Thorsons Publishers Limited, 1985.

CHOTKOWSKI, L A., MD, FACP. "What's New in Medicine: More Than 250 of the Biggest Health Issues of the Decade." Santa Fe, NM: Health Press, 1991.

CONNOR, Sonja L., MS, RD., & Connor, William E., MD. "The New American Diet System." NY, NY: Simon & Schuster, 1991.

DEAN, Ward, MD, et al. "Smart Drugs II: The Next Generation." Petauma, CA: Smart Publications, 1993.

"Delicious. Your Magazine of Natural Living." vol/no 1, Jan 1997.

"Does Leptin Trigger Puberty." Science News vol 151, Jan 25, 1997: p 58.

DOLBY, Victoria. "Rise to the Challenge: Reduce Your Cancer Risk with Garlic Protection." Better Nutrition Dec 1996: p 22.

DUKE, James A. Handbook of Phytochemical Constituents of Gras Herbs and Other Economic Plants. CRC Press, 1992.

ELLIOT, Rose & Depaoli, Carlo. "Kitchen Pharmacy." London, England: Tiger Books International Plc, 1994.

"Environmental Nutrition." vol 19/no 11, Nov 1996.

"Environmental Nutrition." vol 20/no 1, Jan 1997: pp 1-8.

"Environmental Nutrition." vol 19/no 12, Dec 1996.

FACKELMANN, Kathleen. "Rusty Organs: Researchers Identify the Gene for Iron-Overload Disease." Science News Jan 18, 1997: pp 46-47.

"FDA Consumer." Nov 1996: pp 4-5.

FORD, Norman D. "Natural Remedies: Techniques for Preventing Headaches and the Common Cold." NY, NY: Galahad Books, 1995.

FOSTER, Steven. "Phytomedicinals: The Healing Power of Plants." Better Nutrition Dec 1996: pp. 44-49.

FREMES, Ruth & Sabry, Dr. Zak. Nutriscope. Stoddart Publishing Co. Ltd, 2nd ed, 1989.

GARLAND, Sara. "The Complete Book of Herbs and Spices." Pleasantville, NY: The Readers Digest Assoc. Inc., 1993.

GROMLEY, James J. "Saturated Fat- From 'Enemy' to Essential: A Balance of Fat is Key." Better Nutrition Dec 1996: p 12.

"Growing Older Eating Better." FDA Consumer Magazine Reprint: Mar 1996.

"Harvard Women's Health Watch." Harvard Medical School Dec 1996 vol IV/no 4.

"Health News." The New England Journal of Medicine Dec 10, 1996.

HEINERMAN, John. "Heinerman's Encyclopedia of Fruits, Vegetables and Herbs." W. Nyack, NY: Parker Publishing Co, 1988.

"Help Build Strong Bones 8 Ways." Consumer Reports on Health, Dec 1996: pp 135, 138-139.

HENDLER, Sheldon Saul, MD, PhD. "The Purification Prescription." NY, NY: William Morrow & Co. Inc., 1991.

HIKINO, H. "Antihepatonic Actions of Ginerals and Diaryihepataroids." Journal of Ethnopharmacology, vol 14, 1985: pp 31-39.

HORTON, Sara K. "Lose Weight and Keep it Off." Journal of Personality and Social Psychology, vol 70, no 1.

"Housecalls." Health Sept 1996: p 128.

JACOBSON, Michael F., PhD, et al. "Safe Food: Eating Wisely in a Risky World." Los Angeles, CA: Living Planet Press, 1991.

JARVIS, D.C., MD. "Arthritis and Folk Medicine." NY, NY: Rinehart and Winston, 1960: pp 40, 54-55.

JARVIS, D.C., MD. "Folk Medicine: An Almanac of Natural Health Care." NY, NY: Galahad Books, 1958.

KEVILLE, Kathi. "Herbs; An Illustrated Encyclopedia." Michael Friedman Publishing Group, Inc., 1994.

KIKUZAKI, Hiroe & Nakatani, Nobuji. "Antioxidant Effects of Some Ginger Constituents." Journal of Food Science, Institute of Food Technologists, vol 58/no 6, 1993: pp 1408-1410.

KURTZEIL, Paula "Taking the Fat out of Food." FDA Consumer July/Aug 1996: pp 7-13.

LALANNE, Elaine. "Eating Right for a New You." NY, NY: Penguin Group, 1992.

LAMM, Steve MD. "Safe, Lasting Weight Loss: Breakthrough Drug Regimen Makes It Possible," p. 9.

LANGER, Steven MD. "When It Comes to Vitamins, 'Cs' Make the Grade." Better Nutrition, Dec 1996: pp 40-43.

LEBER, Max R., RPh, BS, et al. "Handbook of Over-the-Counter Drugs and Pharmacy Products." Berkeley, CA: Celestial Arts Publishing, 1994.

LIEBERMAN, Laurency MRPh. "The Dieter's Pharmacy." NY, NY: St. Martin's Press, 1990.

"Low- Fat Diets: Moderation and 'Good' Foods Are the Key." UT Lifetime Health Letter Apr 1995: p 7.

"Manganese." Better Nutrition Dec 1996: p 58.

MARIANI, John F. "The Dictionary of American Food and Drink." NY, NY: Hearst Books, 1994.

MCLEOD, Kate. "Stepping Up to healthy Living." Health pp 105-108.

MINDELL, Earl, RPh, PhD. "Earl Mindell's Anti-Aging Bible." NY, NY: Simon & Schuster, 1996.

MORGAN, Brian L.G., PhD. "Nutri- Tips." Stamford, CT: Longmeadow Press, 1991.

NAVARRO, Concepcion M. 'Free Radical Scavenger and Anti- hepatotoxic Activity of Rosmarinus tomentosus." Planta Medica, Stuttgart: Georg Thieme Verlag vol 59, 1993: pp 312-3114.

"Novel Antioxidants May Slow Brain's Aging;" Science News Jan 25, 1997: p 53.

"Nutrition Action Health Letter." Center for Science in the Public Interest. Jan/Feb 1997.

"Nutrition and Your Health: Dietary Guidelines for Americans." U.S. Department of Health and Human Services and U.S. Department of Agriculture Dec 1995.

"Olestra and Other Fat Substitutes (Revised)." FDA Backgrounder Nov 28, 1995: pp 1-2.

PAPAZIAN, Ruth. "Should You Go on a Diet." FDA Consumer Magazine May 1994.

PARSONNET, Mia MD. "What's Really in Our Food." NY, NY: Shapolsky Publishers, Inc., 1991.

PEARSON, Durk and Shaw, Sandy. "The Life Extension Companion." NY,NY: Warner Books, Inc., 1984.

PERCHELLET, Jean-Pierre, et al. "Inhibition of DMBA- Induced Mouse Skin Tumorigensis by Garlic Oil and Inhibition of Two Tumor- Promotion Stages by Garlic and Onion Oils." Nutrition and Cancer vol 14/no 3-4, 1990: pp 183-193.

"Prevention Magazine's Complete Book of Vitamins and Minerals," Wings Books and Rodale Press, Inc., N.Y., NY, 1988: pp. 134-137, 348, 372, 383.

"Prevention's Healing With Vitamins," Ed. of Prevention Magazine Health Books. Emmaus, PA Rodale Press, Inc., 1996.

SANTAMARIA, L et al. "Chemoprevention of Indirect and Direct Chemical Carcinogenesis by Carotenoids as Oxygen Radical Quenchers." NY, NY: Annals of the New York Academy of Sciences; 1988: pp 584-596.

SOMER, Elizabeth, MA, RD. "Food and Mood." NY: Henry Holt and Co., 1995: p 16.

SRINIVAS, , Leela, et al. "Tumerin: A Water Soluble Antioxident Peptide from Turmeric (Curcumalonga)." Archives of Biochemistry and Biophysics vol 292/no 2, Feb 1992: pp 617-623.

SRIVASTAVA, K.C. and Mustafa, T. "Ginger (Zingiber Off Icinale) in Rheumatism and Musculoskeletal Disorders." Medical Hypothesis vol 39, 1992: pp 342-348.

STEINMAN, David: "Diet for a Poisoned Planet," NY, NY: Harmony Books, 1990.

STERNBERG, S. "Can Selenium Ward Off Deadly Cancers?" Science News Jan 4, 1997: p 6.

"Tea for Two: Less Cancer, Less Heart Disease." Consumer Reports on Health Dec 1996: pp 135, 138-139.

"Walking for Exercise and Pleasure." The President's Council on Physical Fitness and Sports 1994: pp 2-4, 11.

WEBB, Denise, PhD, RD. "Foods For Better Health: Prevention and Healing of Diseases." Lincolnwood, IL: Publications International, Ltd., 1995.

"Weight Loss Drugs." New England Journal of Medicine Dec 31, 1996: p 7,

WELLS, Valerie "Think Thin." San Francisco, CA: Chronicle Books, 1992.

WERBACH, Melvyn R., MD. "Nutritional Influences on Illness," A Source Book of Clinical Research. New Canaan, Conn: Keats Publishing, Inc., 1987.

"Working Out the Facts: The Truth Behind Ten Common Myths." Consumer Reports Dec 1996; pp 48-49

ZERDEN, Sheldon "The Best of Health: The 101 Best Books." NY, NY: Four Walls Eight Windows, 1989.

Emily's
Vinegar
Diet
Book

90-DAY
MONEY-BACK
GUARANTEE

❑ YES! Please rush _____ additional copies of Emily's Vinegar Diet Book and my FREE copy of the bonus booklet *"The Incredible Magic of Honey and Vinegar For Healing, Health and Weight Loss!"* for only $12.95 plus $3.98 postage & handling. I understand that I must be completely satisfied or I can return it within 90 days for a full and prompt refund of my purchase price. The FREE gift is mine to keep regardless. *Want to save even more?* Do a favor for a close relative or friend and order two books for only $20 postpaid.

I am enclosing $ _____ by: ❑ Check ❑ Money Order (Make checks payable to James Direct, Inc.)

Charge my credit card Signature _____

VISA MasterCard discover AMEX

Card No. _____ Exp. date _____

Name _____

Address _____

City _____ State _____ Zip _____

Mail To: JAMES DIRECT, INC. • PO Box 980, Dept. VB104 Hartville, Ohio 44632
http://www.jamesdirect.com

✂ please cut here - - - - - - - - - - - - - - - - - - -

Use this coupon to order "Emily's Vinegar Diet Book" for a friend or family member -- or copy the ordering information onto a plain piece of paper and mail to:

Emily's Vinegar Diet Book
Dept. VB104
PO Box 980
Hartville, Ohio 44632

Preferred Customer Reorder Form

Order this...	If you want a book on...	Cost...	Number of Copies...
The Magic of Hydrogen Peroxide	An Ounce of Hydrogen Peroxide is worth a Pound of Cure! Hundreds of health cures, household uses & home remedy uses for hydrogen peroxide contained in this breakthrough volume.	$9.95	
The Vinegar Anniversary Book	Completely updated with the latest research and brand new remedies and uses for apple cider vinegar. Handsome coffee table collector's edition you'll be proud to display.	$9.95	
The Magic of Baking Soda	*Plain Old Baking Soda A Drugstore in A Box?* Doctors & researchers have discovered baking soda has amazing healing properties! Over 600 health & Household Hints. *Great Recipes Too!*	$9.95	
Amish Gardening Secrets	You too can learn the special gardening secrets the Amish use to produce huge tomato plants and bountiful harvests. Information packed 800-plus collection for you to tinker with and enjoy.	$9.95	
Any combination of the above $9.95 items qualifies for the following discounts...		**Total NUMBER of $9.95 items**	

Order any 2 items for: $15.95

Order any 3 items for: $19.95

Order any 4 items for: $24.95

Order any 5 items for: $29.95

Order any 6 items for: $34.95 and receive 7th item FREE

Any additional items for: $5 each

FEATURED SELECTIONS		Total COST of $9.95 items	
Emily's Vinegar Diet	This is the easy-to-follow diet you have been waiting for! It helps you lose weight without counting calories or being hungry. This time, you'll keep the weight off - for life!	$12.95	
Hydrogen Peroxide Formula Guide	FINALLY...No more guesswork! Step-by-step instructions and specific measurements for hundreds of amazing hydrogen peroxide uses. Learn how to use hydrogen peroxide to clean your home, balance pH soil levels, use as a home remedy or beautify your life! It is all here!	$19.95	
Vinegar Formula Guide	This one-of-a-kind, ground breaking book gives you exact formulas and measurements for ALL of your vinegar applications! In it you'll find step-by-step, easy-to-use instructions for home health remedies, cleaning projects and more!	$19.95	
The Cinnamon Book	Research studies have found this amazing spice is loaded with health benefits. Find out how cinnamon can be used in treating common (and not so common) conditions such as diabetes, obesity, arthritis, high cholesterol and a host of other ailments.	$19.95	
Order any 2 or more Featured Selections for only $10 each...		**Postage & Handling**	$3.98*
		TOTAL	

90-DAY MONEY-BACK GUARANTEE

*** Shipping of 10 or more books = $6.96**

Please rush me the items marked above. I understand that I must be completely satisfied or I can return any item within 90 days for a full and prompt refund of my purchase price.

I am enclosing $_____ by: ❑ Check ❑ Money Order (Make checks payable to James Direct Inc)

Charge my credit card Signature _____

Card No. _____ Exp. Date _____

Name _____ Address _____

City _____ State _____ Zip _____

Telephone Number (_____) _____

❑ Yes! I'd like to know about freebies, specials and new products before they are nationally advertised. My email address is: _____

Mail To: **James Direct Inc.** • PO Box 980, Dept. A1405 • Hartville, Ohio 44632
Customer Service (330) 877-0800 • *http://www.jamesdirect.com*

©2016 JDI A253IM

THE MAGIC OF HYDROGEN PEROXIDE

Hundreds of health cures & home remedy uses for hydrogen peroxide. You'll be amazed to see how a little hydrogen peroxide mixed with a pinch of this or that from your cupboard can do everything from relieving chronic pain to making age spots go away! Easy household cleaning formulas too!

THE VINEGAR ANNIVERSARY BOOK

Handsome coffee table edition and brand new information on Mother Nature's Secret Weapon – apple cider vinegar!

THE MAGIC OF BAKING SODA

We all know baking soda works like magic around the house. It cleans, deodorizes & works wonders in the kitchen and in the garden. But did you know it's an effective remedy for allergies, bladder infection, heart disorders... *and MORE!*

AMISH GARDENING SECRETS

There's something for everyone in *Amish Gardening Secrets*. This BIG collection contains over 800 gardening hints, suggestions, time savers and tonics that have been passed down over the years in Amish communities and elsewhere.

EMILY'S VINEGAR DIET

This easiest diet ever helps you lose pounds and inches, and keep them off! With a tonic of apple cider vinegar and honey there is no confusing calorie counting, food restrictions or expensive supplements. Increase your energy level while the pounds melt away. See how to use the "magic" of thermogenesis to be thinner, look younger and feel more vigorous – without depriving yourself of the foods you love!

HYDROGEN PEROXIDE FORMULA GUIDE

This unique book lists hundreds of home remedy, gardening and cleaning uses for peroxide along with exact measurements and instructions for each use. No mistakes and no guesswork.

VINEGAR FORMULA GUIDE

Studies have shown vinegar to be effective at not only cleaning and disinfecting, but also as a natural home remedy for conditions such as lowering cholesterol, fighting disease, easing arthritis, improving circulation and more! Now learn the exact formulas and measurements for EACH home remedy and cleaning project in a concise, easy-to-read format! No more guesswork!

THE CINNAMON BOOK

Cinnamon is rich in natural healing properties such as being an anti-oxidant, anti-inflammatory, anti-coagulant, anti-microbial, anti-parasitic, anti-tumor – just to name a few! Find out how cinnamon can be used to fight everything from simple cuts and scrapes to chronic health condition, safely and naturally!

* Each Book has its own FREE Bonus!